CLEANENOUGH

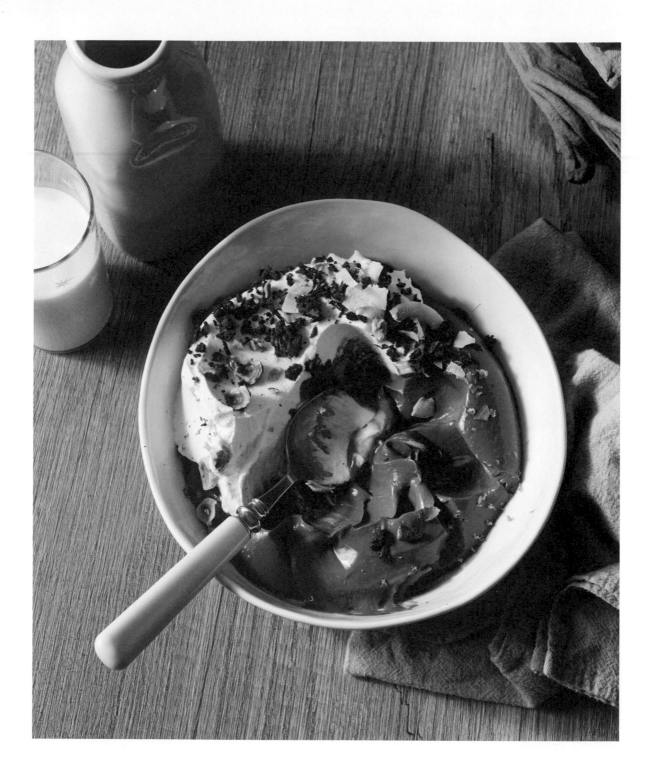

CLEANENOUGH

Get **BACK TO BASICS**
and Leave **ROOM FOR DESSERT**

KATZIE GUY-HAMILTON

THE EXPERIMENT

NEW YORK

The Experiment, LLC | 220 East 23rd Street, Suite 600, New York, NY 10010-4658 | theexperimentpublishing.com

The Experiment's books are available at special discounts when purchased in bulk for premiums and sales promotions as well as for fund-raising or educational use. For details, contact us at info@theexperimentpublishing.com.

Library of Congress Cataloging-in-Publication Data

Names: Guy-Hamilton, Katzie, author.
Title: Clean enough : get back to basics and leave room for dessert /
  Katzie Guy-Hamilton; foreword by Habib Sadeghi, DO.
Description: New York : Experiment, [2019] | Includes index.
Identifiers: LCCN 2018017237 (print) | LCCN 2018019118 (ebook) | ISBN
  9781615195077 (ebook) | ISBN 9781615194902 (cloth)
Subjects: LCSH: Cooking. | Health. | LCGFT: Cookbooks.
Classification: LCC TX714 (ebook) | LCC TX714 .G889 2019 (print) | DDC
  641.5--dc23
LC record available at https://lccn.loc.gov/2018017237

ISBN 978-1-61519-490-2
Ebook ISBN 978-1-61519-507-7

Cover and text design by Sarah Smith
Food styling by Keren Hazan and Katherine Sacks

Manufactured in China
First printing January 2019
10 9 8 7 6 5 4 3 2 1

In memory of my uncle Robbie, Robert McKelvie, the hardest-working man I have ever known. His generosity and selfless acts of love through food tie us together and have been a guiding light in creating Clean Enough. His encouragement to drive forward yet find balance is an everlasting gift. While we may no longer be drinking wine or prepping dinner together, I feel honored to take on the role of making sure that the dinner table will always be a safe place for people to come as they are.

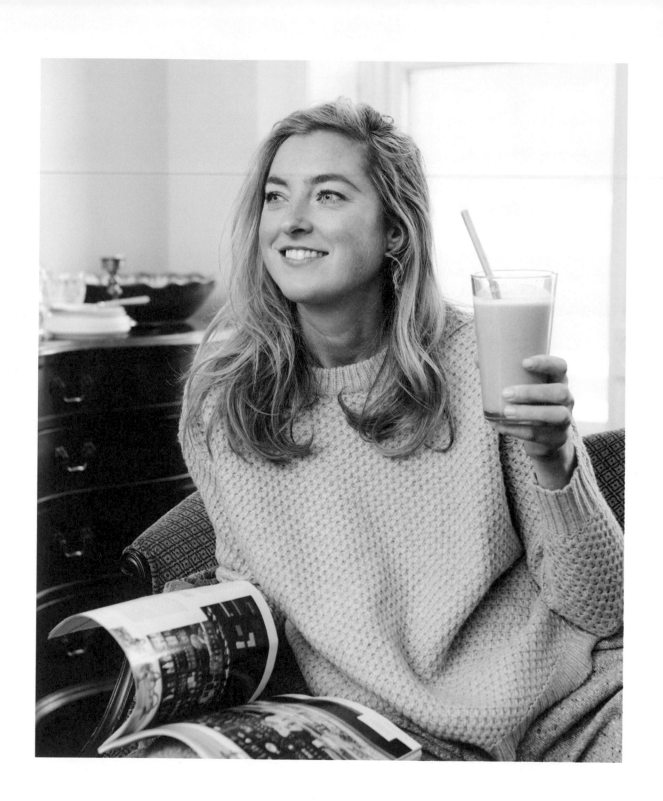

CONTENTS

I. CLEAN

II. ENOUGH

A Taste of Joy

As a physician of integrative medicine, I see patients with complex conditions from all over the world. Because the internet provides so much information these days, it's not uncommon for them to report to me that they're currently taking more than thirty exotic herbs and superfoods, often several times a day. Some have even been on these self-prescribed, complicated nutrition regimens for years prior to getting sick and can't understand how illness could have developed when they were eating all the "right" foods.

In the last several years, I've noticed that whenever a person gets sick, the first thing he or she wants to focus on is their diet. From a certain perspective, I understand this. Changing one's diet can be a powerful way to take an active role in your own healing process and regain some sense of control over your life. On the other hand, while nutrition and supplements can be a valuable support in any patient's treatment plan, those are never the center of it. I can attest to this fact through my own healing from cancer over twenty years ago.

Still, it's very hard for some patients to resist the urge to measure everything they eat, making sure it's organic, non-GMO, free-range, pasture-raised, sustainably farmed, hormone free, sprouted, and certified by all the appropriate agencies. In short, their path to healing has turned eating into a joyless chore that only adds more stress to their lives.

What they've forgotten is that the greatest force for healing is already inside us: joy. It's our ability to feel expansive emotions like love, excitement, gratitude, and connection. When we feel emotions like these, thousands of chemical changes happen in an instant that do everything from improving circulation to speeding wound healing to boosting immune function. Even so, most of us don't have these experiences nearly enough—if at all—in our hectic, workaday lives.

Katzie Guy-Hamilton, in her exuberant work and light-filled person, embodies this deeper understanding of the real mechanisms for well-being and healing. How you feel about your food, and how you make it, matters. As she illustrates in *Clean Enough*, the nutritive power of what we eat isn't black or white, clean or unclean. The occasional slice of her Grandma's Chocolate-Chocolate-Chocolate Cake or ice cream sandwich will do more good for your body than striving to exist on boring salads and bitter green smoothies alone. Many of my patients don't realize this: They grow frustrated when tracking the macronutrients of every meal, doing yoga, meditating, and eating an all-organic diet doesn't make them well. Missing from their menu is joy, the greatest healing prescription any of us can write for ourselves.

Clean Enough overflows with this soul-medicine. Its incredible recipes are as healthy as they are delectable, reminding you that it's okay to not sweat the small stuff like an ice cream sandwich or licked-clean bowl of chocolate pudding. In sharing her own journey to living Clean Enough, she asks the thought-provoking questions about what a healthy diet and lifestyle mean to you—and what you could add to your plate to bring you more joy. These foods—practical and easy to make; with an emphasis on depth of flavor and fresh, wholesome ingredients—will fill you with the perfect amount of mindfulness, taste, and pleasure; and they'll leave you reassured that you are, now and always, more than enough.

—DR. HABIB SADEGHI,
author of *The Clarity Cleanse*

INTRODUCTION

My mission is simple: to live and inspire others to be Clean Enough. You are enough, just as you are, and the pursuit of perfection is a wasted one. *Clean Enough* is here to help establish with confidence that simple fact about you, hopefully saving you some time that you can use instead to experience more of life's joys. Being Clean Enough requires some effort, learning, and patience—it's what I would call good work. Nurturing your body with whole foods presents a host of benefits, one of which is *food freedom*. To me, this means the ability to be all-inclusive, knowing that at a baseline you have the confidence and know-how to properly feed yourself food made from real ingredients, not packages. You will know how to approach food from a standpoint of vitamins and minerals; of heartiness, depending on your hunger and energy needs; of flavor, feeding cravings the wholesome way; and of variety, as in there are endless possibilities with the ingredients that Mother Nature has generously provided. Let's not forget simplicity, as living Clean Enough does not have to be complicated and is basic in its nature. In its purest essence it encourages eating a wide array of vegetables, fruits, grains, nuts, and seeds prepared in a flexible range from raw salads to lightly sautéed, roasted, stewed, and pureed vegetables, and to nourishing legumes and grains. These are unequivocally the foundation to anyone's healthy diet. The mix-ins and additions, unique to you, will allow you to access your optimum health. Being able to care for oneself is an everlasting skill and tool that, once acquired, cannot be unlearned. This will help you start living intuitively, in essence knowing what, when, and how much your body needs at any given time. This includes congee as well as cookies.

Clean and wholesome foods have allowed me to stop demonizing treats, and this book is here to argue the case for you to do so, too. Rather than write a glass castle guide to eating perfectly clean, an unreachable goal, or the sugar-laden half story, I thought I would keep it real. Relying on my background as both a trained pastry chef and a certified health coach, I am presenting you with a variety of tools and recipes to inspire you to eat clean foods. Foods that can be used for both a state of healing and/or graduating you to a higher state of *being*. When you've had enough of clean and the occasion calls for it, take a trip to the sweet side. Not only will you acquire achievable and long-lasting skills in the dessert-making department, developing a unique ability to surprise and delight your community, but you will understand more fully the chemistry, feel, flavor, and aesthetics of your ingredients.

In this book are a lot of stories. I love telling them, painting a picture of ongoing curiosity and my quest for balance. I have and will continue to put in the work right along with you. Many of the recipes show (and honor) how other cultures feed and heal themselves, with spices, purees, and other preparations. This is the story of how I went from being a pastry maven to a kale queen and found balance somewhere in between. My secret? Loving myself for being Clean Enough.

MY STORY

I grew up in Worcester, a small city right in the middle of Massachusetts. A melting pot of cultures, food, and quaint New England neighborhoods. My mom, Janet, is a magenta lipstick–wearing silver fox, hailing from Halifax, Nova Scotia. Her artistic sass fueled my creativity, imagination, and adventurous spirit. My dad, William, was born and raised in Worcester. A bottomless well of historical knowledge, he was into healthy food long before I would accept carrot sticks and celery as a snack and not punishment. My older sister, Rebecca, is a nurse and an athletic force to be reckoned with. She will care for sick patients for thirteen hours straight and hike the Presidential Traverse the following day. My older brother, Matthew, has been my ultimate inspiration. The most driven person I know, he has unknowingly helped me harness my passions in a focused and strategic manner, while still being free.

I had a pretty idyllic childhood experience for a creative spirit like mine: tree-lined streets, flashlight tag, lemonade stands, and encouraging neighbors supporting my various business endeavors. Before I knew what a CV was, I drafted one, sealed it in page protectors, and thumbtacked it to trees throughout the neighborhood. Offering a variety of services that included child, pet, and house care, I did not discriminate.

My first real job was behind the register at George's Fruit and Produce. George's was a Worcester landmark: It boasted fruit, produce, an incredible cheese counter, a deli, and an ice cream shop. I learned about persimmons, sold cheese, and used the space as a testing ground for my newly discovered sweet obsession. I would come in with a pie and request that people try it, watching them carefully for approval.

I knew then that I wanted wholeheartedly to become a pastry chef, feeling lucky enough to have realized a true passion. I drove forward determined to pursue the craft, terrifying my parents that I was choosing to enter into the archaic world of restaurants. My mother told me that *I'd better be successful*—egging me on to do something big.

Enrolling in the French Culinary Institute in New York City was the best decision I could have made, for it gave me an education in the building blocks of great baking. While in school, I began an externship with Deborah Racicot at Gotham Bar and Grill, spending my days making anglaise and chiboust and my evenings chopping cases of rhubarb and learning some of my favorite desserts to this day. Most important, Deborah understood the importance of craveability in presentation: fresh petite apple cider doughnuts, whipped apple cream, and caramel ice cream swirled with something off center, all the while keeping an artistic lens on her plates.

During the summer before graduation from culinary school, I visited the West Coast in hopes of meeting Sherry Yard at the famed Spago in Beverly Hills. Part of Wolfgang Puck's empire, Sherry was the woman at the sweet helm of it all, serving *Kaiserschmarren* to the Hollywood elite while building lasting relationships with farmers, ensuring them stability in exchange for the best figs in Southern California. I cold-emailed her for weeks until she responded. As luck had it, I swiftly returned to New York to finish school before moving to the West Coast for the chance to be a pastry chef at one of my dream restaurants with my dream mentor, Sherry herself.

Spago taught me everything about delicious produce, desserts, hard work, and what a multifaceted organization looks like. A stint in London got me hooked on British desserts, which ultimately led me to the Breslin at the Ace Hotel. I have no idea how I managed to run a pastry department in a hotel, but I definitely dug in, with an amazing chocolate syllabub recipe developed as a result. The next step was the Grand Hyatt at Grand Central, where I managed a staff of professionals on average three times my age, and on weekends finagled the opening of a restaurant with friends in Louisville, Kentucky—RYE on Market, it was called, and it was where I spent my Saturdays and Sundays making buckets of Banana Luscious chocolate pudding. I checked off my bucket list joining a reality television show when I entered *Top Chef: Just Desserts* in 2011. This platform led me to be tapped for Max Brenner, where the CEO, Sam Borgese, was preparing to reopen the company's franchise plans into new markets.

Max Brenner brought me around the world multiple times, and with some pretty incredible chocolate milkshake recipes in tow. I began my role on a world tour with Sam, during which we visited the Philippines, Japan, Korea, Australia, Israel, Singapore, China, and Russia, all in thirty days. I wore many hats, visiting and establishing new markets, doing all of the company's research and development, from chocolate sundaes to macaroni and cheese. As a tall blonde female chef, I was Max Brenner's international brand ambassador. I trained new market teams, did ingredient sourcing in new markets, acted as a traditional food and beverage director . . . did I leave anything out? Plate was full.

Over the years, my desire to learn about wellness intensified. The world travel and constant testing of sweets was an arduous undertaking. I felt as if I were on a hamster wheel without any real tools to help sustain me. I wasn't willing to give up, which led me to enroll in the Institute of Integrative Nutrition (IIN) with the goal of obtaining more healthful culinary skills. Ultimately, IIN taught me more: how to approach sustainable lifestyle changes for both myself and others with a spirit of curiosity and openness.

I took a closer look at what I was putting in my body by choice to help me deal with and balance what I was putting in my body out of obligation for my job. I paid attention to how food was really making me feel, what gave me energy, what made my mood balanced and my waistline consistent (enough). This holistic approach pushed me to take a closer look at my relationships and what I wanted and was willing to contribute. I also considered what made me who I am and if I was leaving space for those interests to be a part of my life, specifically my more spiritual pursuits. My relationship to my job was also examined, along with its relationship to my worth. This was an ego trip that required a bigger reality check than I could have imagined. Was I really spending the majority of my time just feeding my ego? With food, relationships, lifestyle, and my career? A change was on the horizon—a redirection from living wrong was going to require me to stay strong.

How did I get here? Ultimately, I started the process of change by asking myself what mattered to me most. I knew I wanted to participate in the emerging health landscape, and rather than wander during my hiatus, I became purpose-driven. I took a trip to Nosara, Costa Rica—one of my favorite and energetically vibrant places on earth. The Harmony Hotel, and the creative director Monica Ramos, allowed me to come down to contribute, all the while spending time dedicated to caring for myself with plenty of rest and coconuts. I worked on a wellness concierge program, where we highlighted the many forms of exhaustion along with helpful strategies. *Exhaustion* is an umbrella term for many conditions: from stress to not eating enough nourishing foods, from being overtired and low energy to feeling intoxicated by internal or external forces. I took a deep dive into the menu offerings to understand if they would add vitality, nourishment, or a cleaner approach to a meal, thus creating a meal plan tool that could be used by a hotel guest rather than dictated by a dietitian. This was the ultimate self-guided healing. My workshops were internationally focused, talking about self-care with the hotel's staff which solidified the notion for me that everyone, even healers, need to be reminded to pause.

During this exploratory phase, I began writing, reigniting my love of craft, which led me to write down more of my recipes and to think about what I needed to cook and what others might want to know how to make. Documenting the beginnings of *Clean Enough* was exhilarating, along with my "why" starting to take shape.

Trust the process, I told myself. The thought that I wanted to help people create their Clean Enough started to crystallize, yet I had no idea what the function would be, meditating on being in the flow of an emerging path. At a Women's Chefs and Restaurateurs conference and realized so many of my peers wanted others to be well, too. Who knew? There were people outside of my fitness-fanatic crew who cared about achieving health on their own terms. My artistic, personal, and clean-minded aspirations were all being turned on: Express your sweet talent, make time for relationships, eat and be well. The next thing I knew, Equinox came knocking and I dove in, dedicated to a both diet-agnostic and holistic approach to health and performance.

Sharing the concept Clean Enough is my truth. Working in high performance luxury fitness, I still keep bars of dark chocolate at my desk, and my weekends are sprinkled with fresh pies and ice cream. Seeing both extreme sides of the equation, both restriction in wellness and unhinged indulgence in hospitality, has been vital in understanding and developing this strategy that ultimately is unique to every individual. My curiosity paired with a willingness to keep at it, always asking why, has no endpoint. Thus far, it has led me from cookie-scraps scrounging as a young pastry chef, all the way through many personal and professional sweet adventures, to eating too green and clean, ultimately landing somewhere in between, reinforcing an authentic appreciation for that roadside ice cream stand on a hot July day equal to my mornings started with hot water and lemon.

YOUR STORY

Before you get in the kitchen, let's talk about *food* but not in the literal sense. I ask you to pause to acknowledge the elements that make up your universe, that feed you, but that are often ignored and just as crucial as what you physically eat. As you explore the wide array of simple clean recipes, getting acquainted with or reawakening your ability to feed yourself the rainbow of colors and flavors, chew on what feeds your world. Having a well-rounded understanding of food in more inclusive terms will help you in developing your personal mission statement of Clean Enough.

So I ask you, dear reader. How do you feel when well? *Wellness* may be a hot-button word right now, but that feeling of balance and calm—whatever that means to you—will never go out of style. In my experience, the answer lies in figuring out your own personal wellness strategy with a dose of forgiveness, your Clean Enough.

You may also be starting from a place of "vegetables and whole foods are boring." Or "I don't know how to incorporate more color and vitamins into my day; can someone show me how it can make sense?" You may already know your way around the produce aisle and are looking for more inspiration, maybe a little perspective and flexibility, ready to go from Clean to Enough.

Take as much as you want and leave the rest as your Clean Enough unfolds. For some it may mean simply committing to a salad a day, and for others to be inspired to take a deep dive into Luxury Granola, Bibimbap, or Celery Root and Jicama Salad, or mastering meringue.

With this framework, you can build in small actions that honor your values and support your daily reality, thereby adding energy to your everyday, no matter how it unfolds. Focusing on habits that support your day will ultimately lead to new outcomes. Is it eating a better postworkout breakfast, such as the Longevity Mushroom Toast with a runny egg and taking a daily break before work breaks you? Accumulated, healthy habits *are* balance. Over time, you establish a dynamic Clean Enough toolbox available for you to maintain or recalibrate any time, in any season.

The recipes will bring you through the seasons *and* your personal seasons. Just as the earth and its bounty come alive in spring, slow down in the fall, and go quiet in the winter, your nutritional needs do the same. As you explore, try to honor the conditions of your body and mind rather than fight them. Let the Zucchini and Spring Pea Machine energize and Midnight Carrots nourish.

These recipes are foundational, so have at it and most of all have fun! And try to not take the broccoli too seriously.

Your Universe Feeds You

Believe it or not, what goes in your mouth is only a small part of what makes you feel great, healthy, grounded, present, mindful, whole, joyous, crappy, heavy, stressed, or distracted. Understanding what affects your well-being outside of nutrition from food is empowering and gives new meaning to Clean Enough.

The recipes in this book are organized into two sections, "Clean" and "Enough." Leading with "Clean" gets your day off to the right start, helps you build your lunch routine, and creates satisfying dinners. They can easily be made for one, two, or more depending on your needs and desire to get ahead. We end with "Enough": best-of-class desserts that are simple, unique, and always sublime. These timeless treats are to be created to share (including your talents). Who really bakes a perfect chocolate cake for themselves, anyway? Use the desserts to elevate a simple meal with a perfect tart or an elegant (clean) feast with a milkshake, or two. There is a dessert for every occasion.

Your emotional health, all directly impacted by the below, lives in your gut, so to get the most out of what you eat, try to be curious about the big picture.

Ready to begin? Start by asking yourself a few questions about the obligations in your life and their relationship to your available time, as well as to your passions, talents, and taste preferences. Admit to yourself what your go-to is when stressed, triggered, and overwhelmed.

CAREER

We all spend a lot of time working. The majority of our day is spent being on and executing. Take a moment and think about what you "do." Does it excite you—light a flame—or does it tire you? All things considered, are you generally looking forward to spending your day how you do? Are you growing as a person?

Now, I can't tell you how to weigh what you are grateful for, are willing to live with, or need to change, but in naming them you may see how you can change your perspective about your job through adapting or, more radically, finding a new opportunity.

RELATIONSHIPS (FAMILY + FRIENDS)

Your day and how you feel about it is enormously affected not just by how you spend it but by the people you spend it with. Appreciate your relationships, both romantic and otherwise, for without them you are guaranteed to be hungry. Being objective about the people you are emotionally linked to exposes the truth. Oversimplifying this because, well, it is. Be grateful, put in your 100 percent and be honest about what is flat-out not feeding you. Practice forgiveness, even (and especially) with old wounds. Be intentional, building up your inner circle. For they are fed by—and they will feed—you.

MOVEMENT

We all need to move, and I am *not* talking about moving in a state of chronic stress which is not a version of physical activity that can offer focus and a mindful release of tension. Movement doesn't need to be daunting. You do not have to be training for a marathon (but if you are, all the power to you). Physical activity is figuring out the kind of movement that you enjoy, that you look forward to and you can make a habit out of. Doing exercise that your body rejects is a study in the art of the unsustainable. Some of us work better with a trainer or buddy for accountability, whereas others eagerly get themselves onto a tennis court every morning and serve a bucket of balls solo. At the end of the day you are the master of what and how you move.

Refrain from letting yourself be deterred by not being great at something right away. Like making the Pan di Spagna for the first time, physical skills are built by repetition.

SLOW SELF-CARE

Self-care comes in many forms and I encourage everyone, even the most gifted healers and busiest high-performer, to do more of it. Be it turning your phone off at night, talking a walk by yourself once a week, saying Enough when you really just need some greens. These are all forms of self-care. They can be as highbrow as a retreat to Italy or as accessible as an Epsom salts bath at home. Whatever it is, whatever the amount of time, the slowdown itself is necessary to maintaining your achievements. These not only help with the digestion of your clean food, but they help you make better clean food choices and help you tap into what your body intuitively needs from food.

GROUNDING PRACTICE

Building and maintaining a spiritual practice does not require you to belong to an organized religion. Spirituality is both a practice and a feeling: a sense of love, home, community, and security that may or may not happen in a place of worship or within a specific spiritual text. It's about connecting with something that's bigger than you. Use that mind-set to stabilize your response mechanism, perspective, and motivation in the world.

It is fair to note that meditation was key to developing my spiritual practice. I study and meditate on The Foundation for Inner Peace's *A Course in Miracles* and am committed to a perspective of love, regardless of the test.

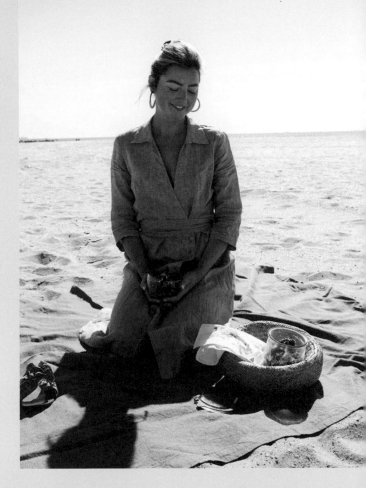

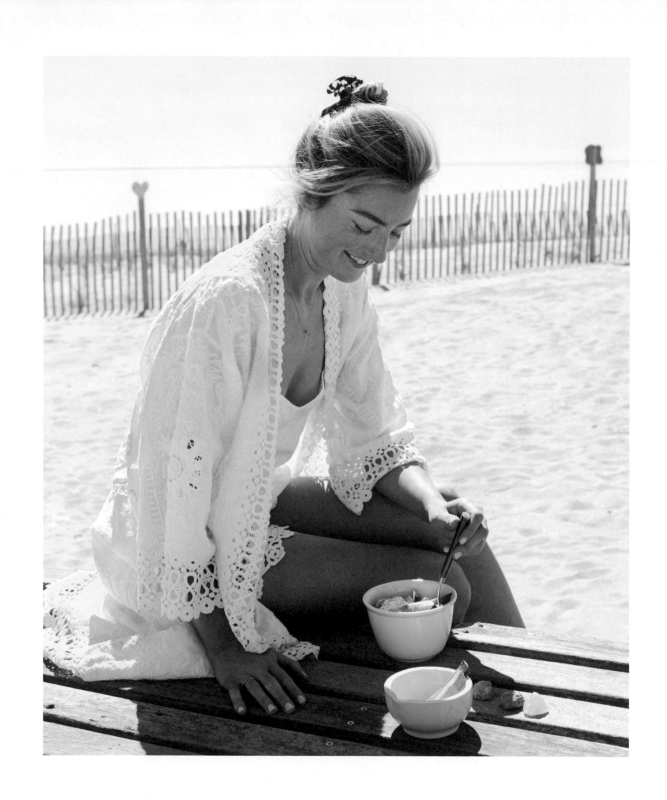

I
—

CLEAN

Why Clean?

You are what you eat and, rather than ignoring this reality, it's time to embrace it. Whole foods, free of preservatives and rich with vibrant color, charge up the body with nutrients for sustained energy, allowing you to look, feel, and truly *be* your best. Yet eating "clean" doesn't mean being afraid of food and subsisting off carrot sticks. Life is best when it is Clean Enough, seeking out the right whole, nourishing foods that work for your unique body in any unique moment.

Food freedom is a big step in appreciating what you are putting in your body. The energy transfers from hand to food to mouth. That means being okay with days when sitting yourself down to a soft-boiled egg and a piece of real whole grain toast with a simple slice of tomato is the best thing that you can for yourself; and other days when you're overcome by a beauty-plate fervor that takes you the extra mile to create an array of the prepared vegetables on top of a batch of dressed greens and rice.

You are going to learn a lot in this section, from salad dressings that are a cinch to make, to the best roasted eggplant you have ever laid your eyes on. Mixing and matching will be a source of power for you here. There are no rules: Have soup for lunch *and* dinner, throw a salad next to the breakfast toast and call it lunch. The variety of nutrients and foods heal, bringing a state of balance and allowing you to tap into your food intuition. When curating these recipes, I drew from an adventurous mind-set: Seek out the cleanest, most authentic food no matter where I am and bring that inspiration home to my kitchen. Many of the staple dishes globally are often (but not always) incredibly healthful.

Clean should and can be simple. What your Clean is, is entirely up to you. I mean this literally, in terms of bioindividuality, which means that every body responds to foods differently. Use these recipes to taste and explore.

CLEAN CUPBOARD

Adding healing spices and understanding the function of ingredients need not be *solely* for the purpose of flushing out and detoxing your system, for the warmth and joy they can bring to the simplest soft scramble or stew is priceless. There is a body-soul connection when it comes to spices. Flavor is met with an array of feelings—grounded, fired up, cleansed, and nourished—as well as function—vitamins, minerals, digestive aids, liver and kidney support, and cognition enhancing, just to name a few.

NOTE ON RECIPES

The recipes in this book are given in household measurements (dry and liquid measuring cups) as well as in grams. Grams indicate ingredients weighed directly on a scale. If weighing liquids on a scale, simply convert the listed *milliliters* to *grams* of the liquid.

All oven temperatures in this book are for a convection oven. If using a conventional oven, increase the recommended temperature by 25°F (15°C)—for example, 300°F (150°C) convection would become 325°F (165°C) conventional—and be sure to rotate the pans during baking for proper heat distribution. Additional baking time (approximately 15 minutes) is often required.

Almond: A source of healthy fats, fiber, and protein, almonds help reduce the inflammation that some people experience with peanut butter. Almonds are naturally sweet and excellent when soaked and blended for nut milks, toasted for salads, added whole and blended into smoothies for texture, flavor, and fiber.

Avocado: There is a reason that we all love this fatty fruit. Avocado adds a creaminess to dressings, smoothies, toasts, and salads. High in potassium, vitamins A, C, E, and K, folate, fiber, and omega-3 fatty acids, which help your body absorb nutrients and remain satiated.

Banana: Potassium-rich, bananas lend creaminess to smoothies and make the most nourishing toast toppings. They are naturally satiating and sweet, and their prebiotic fiber feeds the good bacteria in your digestive system.

Basil: The signature herb of pesto. Basil's pungent aroma and flavor also come with a host of benefits: This herb is antimicrobial, anti-inflammatory, and antioxidant-rich with vitamins and minerals, including vitamin K. Basil is also considered an adaptogen, meaning it combats stress.

Bee Pollen: Mineral-rich bee pollen is a natural antihistamine and fantastic source of energy. Full of lipids and usable carbohydrates, bee pollen is an excellent natural energy source; it is also inflammation reducing and liver cleansing. I like to add this to most of my smoothies.

Black Pepper: When freshly ground, this spice is the no-brainer for anything crusted and seared. It's antimicrobial and aids in digestion, increasing the hydrochloric acid in your gut, and some practices also use black pepper to aid in respiratory issues, such as coughs and colds, where it acts as an expectorant.

Broccoli: All-time. Favorite. Go-To. Steamed. Veggie. In this book, I have it roasted with a dressing;

however, I love it equally steamed in a bowl. An easy cruciferous vegetable that is a nutritional powerhouse full of dietary fiber, vitamins B6 and E, manganese, phosphorus, potassium, copper, iron, and plant protein.

Bragg Liquid Aminos: A fermented soy product that can be used in place of soy sauce (which contains wheat) or tamari (a gluten-free substitute for soy sauce). Comprising amino acids that cumulatively make up complete protein. Liquid aminos also support digestion and tissue growth and repair.

Butternut Squash: Bring on the vitamins. Packed with vitamins A, C, and E, thiamine, niacin, and potassium, squash is satiating like a sweet potato but sans the starch.

Cabbage: A cruciferous vegetable that when fermented into sauerkraut becomes a mealtime probiotic staple. But the humble cabbage can be prepared a million ways, all equally rich in dietary fiber and antioxidants.

Cacao (Raw): Antioxidant-rich and helps normalize blood sugar. Cacao is nothing to shy away from, as raw cacao contains no additives, including sugar. Choosing a high-quality raw powder is essential as it is not alkalized and full of tremendous flavor. Raw cacao is naturally bitter but rich in flavonoids supporting optimal brain function.

Cashew: Not a nut but a seed, cashews are full of vitamin E and healthy unsaturated fats. When blended, they make the creamiest nondairy milk. Also rich in vitamin K and the minerals phosphorus and selenium.

Chestnut: High in fiber and low in carbohydrates, the chestnut is highly unlike its fatty cousins. Its vitamins and minerals, including copper, magnesium, and potassium, keep your bones strong. Chestnuts can easily be found packed in jars; vacuum-sealed, roasted, and peeled; and shell-on ready for roasting.

Chile: Ignite your digestive fire and speed up your metabolism. When fermented, chiles add a sweet and very spicy kick to recipes or on top of soups, toasts, and stews. They also contain high amounts of vitamins A, C, and E.

Cilantro/Coriander Seed: When fresh, the flat-leaf herb cilantro looks similar to parsley and is a great flavoring agent in many cuisines, including Mexican, Thai, and Persian. Packed with vitamins A and K, it can help lower blood sugar, decrease oxidative stress, and regulate anxiety. It is also tapped for regulating your menstrual cycle and overall decreasing inflammation. You will see this herb used in several dishes; don't be afraid to add it to your favorite pesto, salad, toasts, and soup. The dried seed, called coriander, carries the same host of benefits to recipes.

Cinnamon: Cinnamon is like salt and pepper to me. I like it on *a lot* of things, and if you don't already, you will by the end of this book. It's antibacterial, anti-inflammatory, supertasty to a wide variety of palates, and helps with that ever-important blood sugar stabilization. Cinnamon is as calming as it is energizing, and many different cultures incorporate cinnamon from the early years onward: In a pinch, a little steamed milk or cashew milk with honey and cinnamon is as pleasing and calming to a tot as it is to an adult.

Coconut Milk/Oil/Meat: Fear not coconut and its infamous saturated fat! Coconut is a quality source of fat, which we all need in mindful amounts. Its lauric acid helps raise levels of HDL (good) cholesterol.

Coconut has also been found to be antimicrobial and a source of medium-chain fatty acids (MCTs), which supply sustained energy.

Cumin: This spice has historically been used to aid in digestion, which we all know rules your world. My Guacamole loves the addition of cumin, as does the deeply flavorful condiment Rose Harissa.

Dark Leafy Greens: These include spinach, kale, Swiss chard, dandelion greens, chicory, escarole, arugula: all clean sweeps full of folic acid, vitamin C, potassium, magnesium, calcium, and iron. With anti-inflammatory properties, they are detoxifying powerhouses.

Date: My favorite natural sweetener. Fresh dates are whitish green and become brown when dried, obtaining their signature brown sugar–like flavor, juicy texture, and mineral-rich profile. Fresh dates are rarely available outside of specialty markets when in season. High in fiber, potassium, manganese, and copper, these are an instant refined sugar replacement.

Egg: Eggs come in all shapes and sizes as well as quality. *Cage-free* does not denote organic and simply means the chicken was not in a cage. *Free-range* means some access to the outside, but they can be confined to a very small area. *Organic pasture-raised* will signal the highest-quality eggs that you can buy, from chickens fed organic food and allowed to roam freely. I find that the closest thing to a European rich, bright orange egg yolk comes from eggs that are both organic and pasture raised.

Endive: A bitter green cruciferous lettuce that is shaped like a spear, endive is packed with a host of vitamins that aid in metabolism of fat, protein, and carbohydrates, as well as protect your eyesight and reproductive system. It also fights cancer with a high concentration of vitamins A and K, manganese, folate, niacin, and pantothenic acid. This is a perfect sturdy green leaf to roast or grill, as well as to use fresh for salads and as a vehicle for dips and spreads—everything from pesto to Tzatziki to roasting the spears with orange. Everything tastes great on endive.

Extra Virgin Olive Oil: With healthy fats and a spicy bite, extra virgin olive oil, made from cold-pressed olives, is essential for sautéing vegetables, and helps in nutrient absorption of raw foods. With its omega-3 and omega-6 fatty acids as well as polyphenols for brain cognition, you can't go wrong with this source of unsaturated fat gifted from the gods. Choose a high-quality organic oil from the United States, Italy, Spain, or Greece, for use in medium-heat cooking as well as unheated on fresh vegetables, grains, toasts, soups, and salads.

Fennel/Fennel Seed: A digestive aid both in raw and seed form. With a licorice-like flavor, fennel is naturally sweet and warming.

Fig: Another food of the gods, feeding a spiritual soul, figs are rich in fiber, vitamins B6 and K, and such minerals as calcium for bone density and potassium to support low blood pressure. Figs are naturally sticky and sweet without any additives and have been eaten for centuries as both a pleasurable and nourishing food.

Garlic/Black Garlic: One of the original antimicrobial ingredients used for natural healing and a remedy for any viral ailment, garlic is a go-to flavoring agent. Pungent when raw, garlic becomes sweet and mellow when roasted or fermented.

Ginger: Ginger was not originally part of the Western diet, yet we all seem to love the pungent spicy root. Grated into a dressing, marinades, baked goods, granola, smoothies or juice, ginger always adds a kick. Whether this root is pickled or fresh and or piled on top of a stellar bibimbap or congee bowl, or grated into healing tonics and dressings, I find my love for ginger to be akin to that of cinnamon. Ginger is antibacterial, flavorful, and perfect for clearing the mind and digestive system. (Use a Microplane to grate for best results.)

Hazelnut: Beautifully rich and flavorful, hazelnuts when toasted add an intense flavorful aroma to many dishes. Full of healthy fats and fiber, they also contain a high amount of vitamin E, which is essential for health skin and nails.

Himalayan Pink Salt: A natural, unprocessed salt that maintains trace minerals, such as magnesium. Helps regulate hydration as compared to processed iodized salt, which is the culprit behind feeling bloated and dehydrated.

Labne: A strained yogurt cheese made from unsweetened Greek yogurt. The yogurt becomes very tart and thick and is a great spread as well as an ingredient for dips, soups, and so on. High in calcium, low in sugar, and full of probiotics that are good for your digestive tract.

Legumes: These include lentils, gigante beans, black beans, adzuki beans, and chickpeas. Full of dietary fiber, plant protein, vitamins, and minerals, legumes have you covered when it comes to a heart-healthy and strengthening food. They are rich in folate, which supports women's health and is a great blood sugar regulator. Minerals found in sea vegetables, such as kombu, when added to the cooking liquid, aid in the digestion of legumes.

Lemon/Preserved Lemon: Rich in vitamin C, lemons are my go-to for daily morning system cleans and great for your kidneys. I find that lemon helps break down fatty food as well as soothes my stomach for digestion. A standard for bringing out the flavor in food as an accessible source of acid.

Licorice Powder: Licorice holds a special place in my heart. This root has a sweet flavor reminiscent of anise and fennel and can similarly help calm your stomach, reduce stress levels, and aid in the production of healthy mucus. I have the taste for it both in sweet and savory applications.

Maca: A root considered to be an adaptogen, meaning it supports your ability to combat stress and reach a state of balance. Maca balances stress hormones and supports sustained energy. The gelatinized variety is easier on digestion.

Matcha: Superfine ground green tea that is antioxidant-rich and offers a caffeine boost without the crash of coffee. I have a beautiful bag of it I bought in Japan five years ago that I finished while writing this book. Matcha contains L-theanine, an amino acid that contributes to mental relaxation similar to the effects of meditation. A natural energizer that has antihistamine properties and is mineral-rich and soothing.

Mint: A fresh green herb essential in my Pesto and a fantastic addition to brighten up the flavors in salads and toasts.

Mint aids in digestion, decreases bloating, and is naturally cooling and calming. A high antioxidant and a natural anti-inflammatory known to decrease allergy symptoms.

Miso (White): A fermented soybean paste that, while salty, is packed with probiotics. Best used when not boiled, miso is antiviral and gut healing. Chickpea miso is now more widely available for those with soy sensitivity.

Mushroom: Mineral-rich and full of anticancer benefits with just one small mushroom a day. Some mushrooms, such as chaga and reishi, are not often used to cook, but they come imported and dried and have profound benefits for energy, concentration, and cell protection. The fresh section of the grocery store also has a wide variety of mushrooms with diverse benefits and flavor. They are among some of the most healing foods, and I encourage you to try out a little mushroom in place of or in addition to your coffee to see how it makes you feel, as well as to incorporate whole mushrooms into your whole food diet. While I do not advocate anything as a magic wand, the cumulative effects of mushrooms with a healthy diet is something to note.

Mustard: I love mustard powder and seeds for that extra kick in braises and dressing. I could put prepared mustard on anything—though I try to practice self-control for the sake of salt intake and bad habits. Unlike its condiment cousins, mustard lends a lot of flavor sans the calories.

Nutmeg: My go-to on the sweet and savory stuff—yes, nutmeg is as fabulous with any dark green as it is on chocolate mousse, custard tart, brown sugar tart, cookies . . . you name it. I use it as a finishing seasoning as you would finishing salt. A little nutmeg totally changes the memorable factor in a lot of treats. Antibacterial and awesome, this one really cleans up.

Oats: Rich in fiber and a slowly digested carbohydrate, oats are one of the original (though little-known) gluten-free grains that are an energizing and satiating way to start the day or have an energy-rich snack. Rich in fiber and protein, flaked rolled oats are the easiest to prepare, and steel-cut oats are heartier, with a grainier texture and longer cooking time.

Onion: A bitter spicy root in the allium family that is great for digesting fat. Although for some it can cause bloating and crying, be not afraid. The onion is a great base for most meals when sautéed, slowly caramelized, or roasted. Packed with chromium for blood sugar regulation, vitamin C and phytonutrients for healthy cell growth, and quercetin, an anti-inflammatory flavonoid.

Oregano: Oregano is as romantic to me in a shaker at a pizza parlor as it is in a whole bunch freshly plucked from the farmers' market. Can be mixed with olive oil for insanely deliciously grilling. Thought to alleviate many issues, from respiratory tract infections to menstrual cramps and acne, this green herb from the mint family is an excellent rub, salad topper, and soup companion.

Parsley: The classic flat-leaf herb is an excellent detoxifier for your blood and kidneys, aids in digestion, and is a natural diuretic; it is also cleansing as an antimicrobial herb. I put it in most of my herb blends found in salads, such as the Bright Bean Sprout Salad.

Probiotic: Probiotics contain healthy bacteria to support the growth of healthy bacteria in your digestive system. Healthy bacteria results in proper digestion and nutrient absorption. Juice Press's proprietary blend of vegan probiotics called Proviotics are my go-to. I take this in the morning and also add it to my fermented products to help stabilize them in my fridge since I make them at home.

Pumpkin Seed/Pepita: Chock-full of omega-3 fatty acids, protein, fiber, and vitamins and minerals, pumpkin seeds are nutrition and energy powerhouses. They are unique for their zinc content, which supports immunity, and tryptophan, a great natural relaxant and sleep aid.

Radish: A spicy, bitter vegetable that is a brilliant digestive aid. High in vitamin C and low in calories as well as carbs. I love radishes raw on guacamole, on toast, with butter, in salads, and as a snack.

Raw Honey: Raw honey is a natural antihistamine and unrefined sweetener with a unique flavor. Honey varieties vary depending on what type of flowers bees collect nectar from, resulting in a wide range of flavors, from orange blossom to buckwheat. Raw honey has not been treated, leaving all the natural bacteria and minerals and antioxidants intact. Also known for its antifungal properties, raw honey finds its way into many natural beauty products as well as such recipes as the Good as Gold Milk.

Rosemary: A beautiful pine-y herb from the mint family, rosemary has been shown to increase concentration. In essential oil form, I keep it at my desk to catch my midafternoon slump. The essential oils found in rosemary are antifungal, anti-inflammatory, and full of antioxidants, whether applied topically or inhaled as an oil or in cooking.

Rose Water/Rose Petal: Rose is known to reduce inflammation and hyperpigmentation on skin, but it's just as good inside your body. When dried, wild rose petals are incredible added to and served with such condiments as harissa. Rose water, used for Tzatziki, should also be made from wild rose petals and water only, for purity.

Sage: A pungent and velvety leafy green herb with fantastic antimicrobial effects. Sage has been known to support mental concentration and memory retention. With anti-inflammatory and immune-boosting properties as well as high vitamin and antioxidant content, this medical herb has been used for centuries.

Sesame (Seed/ Paste/Toasted Oil): Bursting with texture and intense flavor when toasted, whole sesame seeds are also in za'atar blend and, when ground, make delicious tahini paste. The raw oil is great for neutral cooking at high heat, whereas a small drizzle of the toasted variety adds an intense nutty flavor to dishes as a garnish. Sesame's benefits, in all its forms, include lowering cholesterol, normalizing blood pressure, balancing hormones, and increasing nutrient absorption; it is also host to vitamins and minerals, including manganese and copper. For tahini, I am loyal to the Beirut brand in a clear glass jar with a gold label.

Sourdough: An age-old bread that, when made with high-quality freshly ground wheat, is the thoughtful and digestible choice when enjoying bread. The natural leavening present contains lactic acid, which helps combat the mineral-binding phytic acid present in many whole grain products.

Sumac: A sour, dried spice prevalent in Lebanese cuisine and one of the components of a za'atar spice blend. Sumac helps pump up flavor without having to salt your food heavily. I love this on eggs, soups, yogurt, salads, and legumes. High in antioxidants and helps to control blood sugar.

Thyme: Thyme is a woody, strongly flavored antimicrobial herb used for its antiseptic and antifungal properties. Thyme supports digestion and with its strong aroma has been shown to have mood-boosting properties. The flavor is loved by autumn and winter fruits and vegetables, such as pears, butternut squash, and mushrooms.

Turmeric: An excellent flavor and color additive, in addition to its famed anti-inflammatory properties, turmeric is really as great as they all say it is. That said, it's not a cure-all and can't totally cancel out your trigger— but it will help. A shot of lemon, ginger, and fresh turmeric in the morning really do react well to a just-rested system. It's essential when making a batch of rice, curry, or herb rub. Remember, inflammation is the root of all disease, so go ahead and help yourself deliciously.

Walnut: With omega-3 fatty acids, fiber, and protein, walnuts are a true superfood; when soaked, their soft texture makes them easier to digest than almonds.

Full of manganese and copper, walnuts also contain biotin for healthy hair, skin, and nails.

Za'atar: A mixture of thyme, sesame, and sumac, za'atar is a unique seasoning that I love on top of my salads, toast, and yogurt, as well as for use in marinades. It's traditionally made with an oil base as a jarred liquid condiment, although the recipes here are all referring to the dry spice mix. Savory, sour, and a little smoky, za'atar is something you can truly crave.

DRINK TO YOUR HEALTH

Warm drinks nurture, detoxify, and balance, from one of the simplest acts of self-care, hot water with lemon, to the full healing tonic of Good as Gold Milk. Warm beverages ease digestion, signal elimination, and decrease inflammatory responses.

Cold, blended smoothies are a great way to consume functional macro- and micronutrients in an easy to digest, chew-free, and transportable fashion. Although you may not be inclined to have avocado on your porridge, or kale on your Luxury Granola, they both are medicinal and nutrient-dense foods that can easily be blended into the Green Pow Pow Smoothie. Juices are a fantastic, natural source of vitamins and carbohydrates without the addition of added sugars or energy supplements. They are also a great tool when you don't want a meal and they are better than reaching for a multivitamin from a jar. While I am not a protein-drink-obsessed junkie, having protein in smoothies can further your satiety and fulfill your individual dietary needs. Chia seeds and almonds, just to name a couple, are some of the most readily available plant-based proteins that can be blended into any smoothie, adding healthy fat, fiber, and protein. A bit of fun and function is what I like to bring to all of my potions, with an offering that can be utilized during various times of your day and modified to suit your needs and preferences.

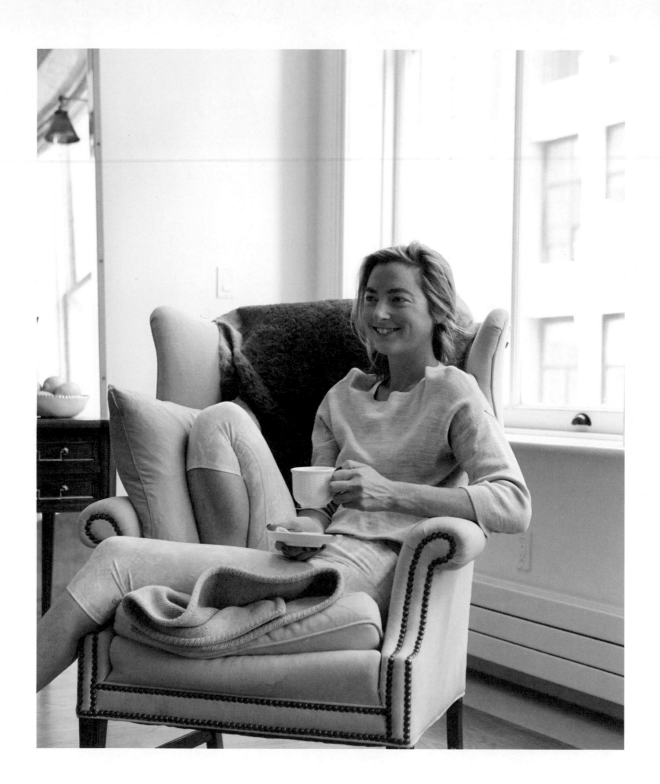

HOT WATER WITH LEMON

To start with the simple (and obvious): the best form of self-care for me starts as soon as I wake up. I drink a glass of water and make myself hot water with lemon. This simple act also comes into play as a soother when I am feeling completely overwhelmed, when I want to snuggle and relax, at the end of a meal, or when I want to meet a friend for an alcohol-free nightcap. Just two ingredients, the humblest you can get, can quickly become a habit that will change your life inside and out. Why? Because lemon has natural antimicrobial properties: it helps ignite digestion, especially with the addition of the warm water; flushes your liver, an organ essential for the removal of toxins; and supports your kidneys' staying free of stones. With a boost of antioxidant-rich vitamin C, this sweet and tart drink has been a remedy for generations for a reason. Besides the direct health benefits, drinking hot water with lemon is a positive habit, a behavior in line with listening abilities and a general awareness, which are the secret to being in a right mind-set and receiving a lot of miracles. You don't have to believe me; just try it.

Makes 1 serving

½ lemon (save the other half of the unjuiced lemon for later)

Scant 1 cup (225 ml) boiling water

1. Juice the lemon half directly into a coffee mug.

2. Tear or, using a vegetable peeler, remove a small strip of zest and place in the mug with the juice. Discard the remaining lemon rind.

3. Pour the boiling water into the mug.

4. Allow the lemon water to cool just enough that you can drink it.

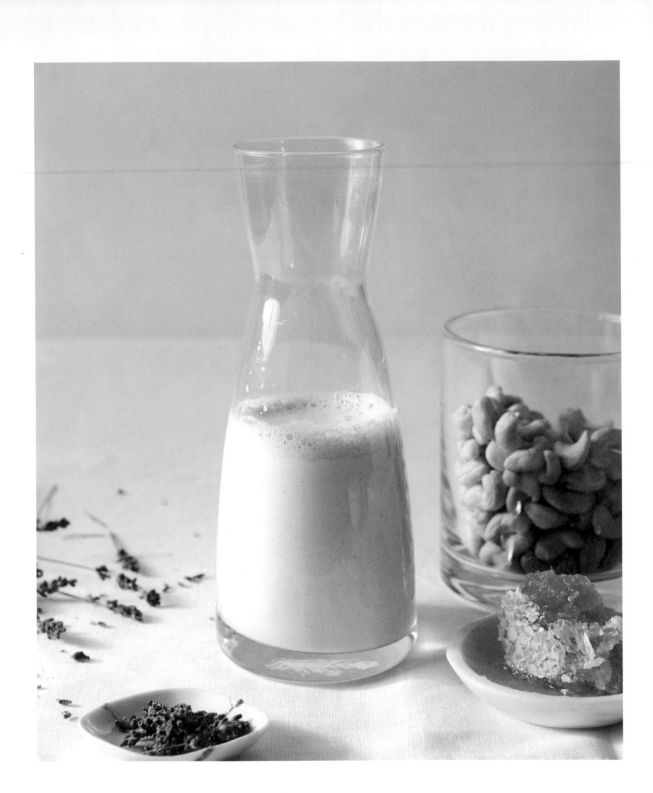

CLEAN ENOUGH

· 12 ·

DESIGNER CASHEW MILK

Creamy and delicious cashew milk is a cinch to make at home, plus it has zero waste. While almond milk has its place in my heart, I have a big issue with the waste that comes with almond milk. Most people do not reuse or compost the heap of strained almond meal that results from the "milking" process. Cashews, on the other hand, are dynamite for the beverage application. Cashews are actually seeds of the cashew fruit, also known as cashew apple, and contain 10 percent starch, which is perfect when making nut milk without any additives. Why? Because nut milk is not actually milk all; rather, it is either all or a portion of a pulverized nut suspended in water, with the natural starch acting as an emulsifier. Cashew milk is packed with healthy fats, vitamin E, and protein. I highly recommend starting your day with a jar of this tossed into your bag with some granola (page 22), or at the ready for a smoothie or smoothie bowl. The lightly scented lavender is so complementary to the creamy cashews that I consider this version my standard cashew base, and it is in fact the base for many drinkable treats to come. Oh, and my mom's dog, Cameron, loves it.

Makes 5 servings

Scant ¾ cup (100 g) raw cashews

2½ cups (600 ml) filtered water

½ teaspoon dried food-grade lavender buds

½ teaspoon raw honey

½ teaspoon vanilla bean paste

⅛ teaspoon Himalayan pink salt

1. Combine the cashews with ½ cup (120 ml) filtered water in a lidded container and allow to soak in the fridge for 3 to 8 hours. In the morning, drain the cashews and discard the soaking liquid.

2. Combine the cashews with the remaining ingredients, including the 2 cups (480 ml) fresh filtered water, in a high-powered blender. Blend on high speed for 1 minute.

3. Store in an airtight container in the fridge for up to 5 days.

VARIATION

Liquirzia Cashew Milk: If you like the naturally sweet flavor of licorice, you will love this twist on cashew milk with the added liver-boosting benefit of raw licorice powder: Simply add ½ teaspoon raw licorice powder to the blender prior to blending.

BANANA NUT SMOOTHIE

This concoction is my personal *pura vida*, meaning "pure life." I find it deeply satisfying when I need a break from the color green and am craving a treat without fully committing to one. This smoothie is full of healthy fats, antioxidant-rich cacao powder, loads of fiber and magnesium, and circulation-boosting cinnamon. When I am looking for a mini-siesta from life, I make this.

Makes 1 serving

1 organic banana, chopped and frozen

About ½ cup (115 to 130 ml) coconut water or water

4 ice cubes

1½ Medjool dates, pitted

1 tablespoon golden flax seeds, ground

1 tablespoon raw almonds

1 tablespoon raw cacao powder

½ teaspoon ground Ceylon cinnamon

1 Proviotic, optional (see Notes)

½ teaspoon gelatinized maca root, optional (see Notes)

1. Combine all the ingredients in a high-powered blender and blend on high speed for 1 to 2 minutes, until smooth and creamy.

2. Pour into a glass and drink immediately.

VARIATION

Make it green (if you must!) by adding a handful of spinach to the blender.

NOTES

Keep your fruit and vegetables prepped and stored weekly in the freezer so that you always have a smoothie available.

Proviotic is simply a vegan probiotic that helps support a balance of healthy bacteria in the small intestine. Probiotics are fed by prebiotic fiber, which bananas contain. I throw the entire capsule into my smoothies before blending.

Maca is a root considered to be an adaptogen, meaning it supports your ability to combat stress and reach a state of balance. A great tool for those who are affected by stress, maca balances and supports sustained energy. The gelatinized variety is easier on digestion.

Add a dusting of ground cinnamon on top for an extra sweet and spicy note.

RUNNER'S JUICE

Naturally sweet and high in nitrates, which increase blood flow and oxygen utilization, beets can help power your long-distance runs. Carrots, pineapple, and orange amp up the energy and flavor and are full of bright phytonutrients, meaning plant-derived vitamins that your body needs. I love bitter juice and tend to process the entire orange, skin on; however, for this recipe you can juice the orange prior to blending.

Makes 1 serving

1 small beet

1 large carrot

¼ cup (40 g) fresh pineapple

Juice of ½ orange

1-inch (2.5 cm) piece fresh ginger

3 cherry tomatoes

1. Process all the ingredients in a juicer, being sure to push all the juice out of the fruit and vegetables, leaving just the fiber behind.

2. Pour into a glass and drink immediately.

CINNAMON CARROT LEMONADE

There is nothing complicated about this juice made with bright, sweet, and juicy flavors. Carrots seem to have fallen by the wayside in favor of green juice, but still hold their place in the realm of fresh juice. The bright orange carrots are a great source of beta-carotene, an antioxidant essential for both eye and reproductive health. The addition of lemon in the carrot juice is what makes it extra tart, yet perfectly balanced by warming cinnamon. Completely unrelated but equally tart, sweetly spiced, and delicious is a juice of plums instead of carrots.

Makes 1 serving

2 large carrots

Juice of 1 lemon

½ teaspoon ground Ceylon cinnamon

1. Juice the carrots using a vegetable juicer. Transfer to a high-powered blender and add the lemon juice and cinnamon.

2. Blend on high speed for 30 seconds, or just to break up any clumps of ground cinnamon.

3. Warm in a heavy-bottomed saucepan to serve hot, or serve over ice.

VARIATION

For a late-summer stone fruit version, replace the carrots with pitted plums, still utilizing a vegetable juicer. Plums will impart a purple hue full of antioxidants.

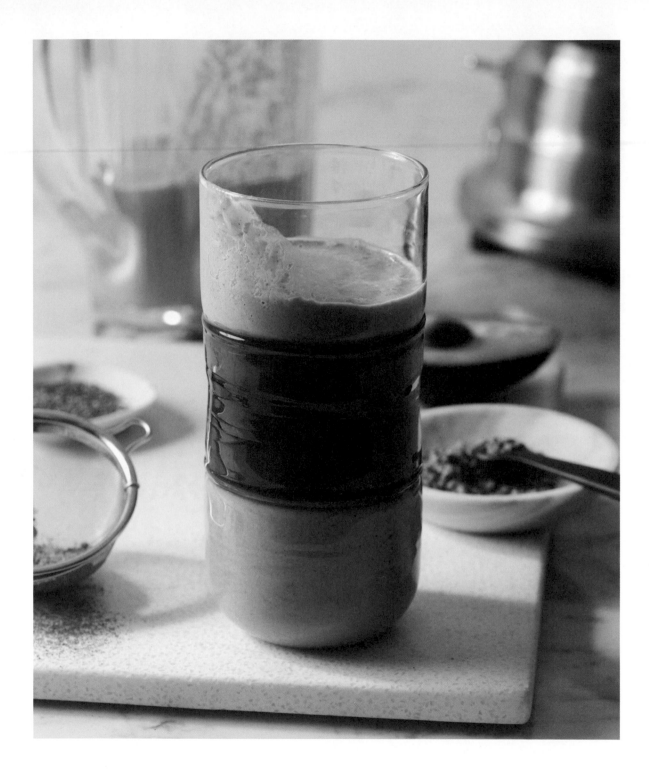

GREEN POW POW SMOOTHIE

When I first started making smoothies, I would make big pitchers of seemingly not delicious brownish-green blends that I would pour into multiple jars and carry around. My game was always: How much kale and spinach can I fit into one jug? This is where the Pow Pow originated and has evolved significantly since then, as I would actually serve this to another human. This smoothie is clean and balanced with fiber, antioxidants, a little matcha kick, healthy fats, and minerals. Matcha's caffeine high and subsequent decline is much smoother than the typical coffee-induced caffeine spike that precedes a sharper decline. When you have a smoothie full of healthy fats like this, it is best keep the sugar low for balanced insulin and digestion.

Makes 1 serving

Large handful of kale, stemmed
(½ cup/20 g)

Large handful of spinach
(½ cup/20 g)

¾ cup (180 ml) Designer Cashew
Milk (page 13)

¼ avocado

4 ice cubes

1 tablespoon chia seeds

1½ teaspoons matcha green tea
powder

1 teaspoon bee pollen

1 tablespoon filtered water, to thin,
optional

¼ teaspoon pine pollen, optional
(see Notes)

1 Proviotic, optional

1. Combine all the ingredients in a high-powered blender and blend on high speed for 1 to 2 minutes, until smooth and creamy.

2. Pour into a glass and drink immediately.

———

NOTES

Frozen kale and spinach work well in this smoothie. Either purchase organic frozen greens or place fresh kale and spinach in bags or glass containers to store in the freezer.

Pine pollen, a powerful herb used in Chinese medicine, is tapped as a nutrient-dense healer and adaptogen, utilized for its claimed anti-inflammatory, endocrine, hormonal, and anti-aging support. If you are prone to allergies and are sensitive to pine (think a Christmas tree), ask before you consume pine pollen!

ROOIBOS CHAI LATTE

I first had this tea when I was living in Chiswick in West London, working at a fine dining restaurant as my own version of study abroad. On my days off I would make rooibos tea and eat Medjool dates while watching the prep school girls across the street belt out love ballads during recess. Rooibos, pronounced *roy-bose* (you are welcome and now can confidently order this tea in public), is a red bush tea from South Africa that is energizing without the addition of caffeine and full of antioxidants. The warming chai spices round out the sweet earthiness of the rooibos. This latte is made with walnut milk, as I feel the nut has a complementary flavor to the tea, but it works just as well with cashew milk.

Makes 3 servings of chai base

BASE

1 cup (100 g) raw walnuts

1⅔ cups (400 ml) filtered water

Juice of 2 oranges

1 tablespoon loose rooibos tea leaves

1 teaspoon ground Ceylon cinnamon

½ teaspoon freshly grated nutmeg

½ teaspoon ground cardamom

½ teaspoon ground ginger, or 1½ teaspoons grated fresh ginger

¼ teaspoon ground cloves

Pinch of freshly ground black pepper

TO SERVE

⅓ cup (80 ml) boiling water per serving

Honey or pure maple syrup, optional

1. Cover the walnuts with the filtered water and place in the fridge for 3 hours or overnight.

2. Combine the walnuts and their soaking water (do not strain) with the orange juice, tea leaves, and spices in a high-powered blender.

3. Blend on high speed for 1 minute.

4. Transfer the liquid to a small saucepan and bring to a simmer for 1½ minutes, stirring.

5. Remove from the heat. Allow the mixture to sit for 3 minutes before straining through a fine-mesh chinois or rounded strainer, almond milk bag, clean coffee filter, or tea strainer, being sure to push out all the liquid, discarding the tea leaves for compost.

6. To prepare a single chai latte: Place generous ½ cup (150 ml) of the chai base in a high-powered blender with ⅓ cup (80 ml) boiling water and blend on high speed to create a froth. Alternatively, you can combine the base with the hot water in a jar and shake to froth or use a cappuccino wand to aerate. Serve with honey or maple syrup, if desired.

VARIATION

Replace the walnuts and filtered water with 2 cups (480 ml) prepared Designer Cashew Milk (page 13), and add to the blender with the orange juice, tea, and spices. Continue to follow instructions from step 3.

GOOD AS GOLD MILK

Unbelievably delicious and nourishing, this medley of spices reduces inflammation and increases digestive fire—besides being just beautiful to look at. Curcumin is the active ingredient in turmeric, and its anti-inflammatory benefits are further activated by the black pepper. The healthy fats found in walnuts further reduce inflammation, with the additional spices supporting circulation, digestion, and natural detoxification of your system. Serve this warm or cold; it is most soothing while warm.

Makes 4 to 5 servings

1 cup (60 g) unsweetened coconut flakes

½ cup (60 g) raw walnuts

2 teaspoons ground turmeric, or 1 tablespoon grated fresh

1 teaspoon ground Ceylon cinnamon

½ teaspoon raw licorice powder

¼ teaspoon freshly grated nutmeg

¼ teaspoon freshly ground black pepper

¼ teaspoon grated orange zest (from ½ orange)

¼ teaspoon scraped vanilla bean seeds

Pinch of Himalayan pink salt

2 teaspoons raw honey or pure maple syrup

1. Combine the coconut flakes, walnuts, and 1½ cups (360 ml) water in a container and place in the fridge for 3 hours or overnight.

2. Combine the soaked nuts (unstrained) with the remaining ingredients in high-powered blender and add 1½ cups + 2 tablespoons (390 ml) water.

3. Blend on high speed for 2 minutes, or until smooth.

4. Strain, using a fine-mesh chinois strainer, being sure to press out all the liquid with a small ladle.

5. To serve warm, heat the strained golden milk in a small pot over medium until just before boiling.

6. Place the hot liquid in a high-powered blender, being sure to secure the lid well. Blend on high speed for 1 minute. Alternatively, use a cappuccino froth wand or a steam wand on an espresso machine.

NOTES

I recommend soaking your walnuts and coconut shreds overnight, but if you are short on time you can pour some boiling water over them and allow them to stand for 10 minutes.

This milk can be made with the Designer Cashew Milk (page 13), replacing the walnut cashew milk with 3 cups + 2 tablespoons (750 ml) prepared cashew milk.

If you do not have a fine-mesh strainer, strain using an almond milk bag, cheesecloth draped in a strainer, or a clean disposable coffee filter.

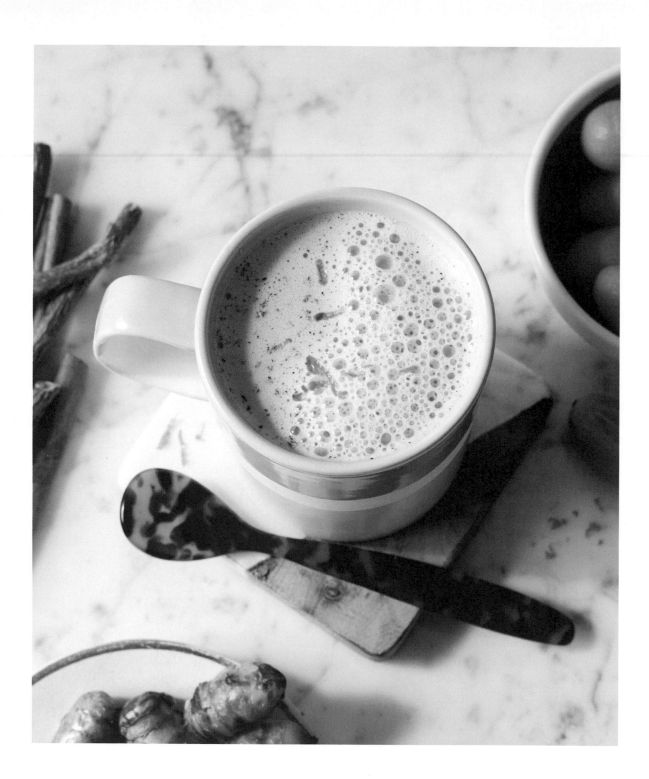

HARMONY BOWLS

Couldn't we all use a bit more harmony in our lives? What could be easier than getting it from nourishing bowl? Perfectly portioned for a hit of nutritional bliss before the day begins, or to feel good at any time, these bowls are a balance of carbohydrate, greens, and protein. Bowls by nature simplify portion control, so have a favorite bowl on hand in a size that suits you. Even with healthful food and a lot of know-how, intentional eating can go off the rails at times; we all, in fact, are human. In those times, I remind myself that there is no such thing as "free food," that nothing should really be consumed with abandon. Redirecting your efforts to the harmony of a single-serving bowl with a simple meal is a useful antidote. The sentiment of having a bit of harmony at mealtime can be utilized any time of day. Feel free to turn recipes not included in this section into your own bowls, layering the good starch, prepared vegetables, greens, and condiments to create your little piece of harmony.

Beginning with all things oats, the porridge, granola, overnight oats, and the smoothie bowl are all excellent sources of morning fuel prior to a workout or as a sustaining feel-good breakfast. For those of the eggier persuasion, pasture-raised organic eggs are shown great care to transform a bowl of spicy radishes, breakfast greens, or melted tomatoes and tahini. Explore your harmony.

LUXURY GRANOLA

The name says it all. Start your day with the best and set the tone for the rest to follow. *No refined sugar added*, crisped with extra virgin olive oil, laced with sweet spices and coconut flakes, kicked up with citrus zest, and made hearty with fancy Sicilian pistachios and almonds, nothing is overlooked. Use the granola on its own for a perfect bowl of energizing carbohydrates and healthy fats. Keep it around for a snack or as a topping on smoothie bowls or your Tahini Banana Bee Toast (page 45).

Makes 12 to 15 servings

Olive oil for pan

Zest of 2 oranges

¾ cup (180 ml) fresh orange juice (from about 2 large navel oranges)

¾ cup (150 g) Medjool dates, pitted

⅔ cup (160 ml) extra virgin olive oil

2 teaspoons Maldon sea salt flakes

1 teaspoon Ceylon ground cinnamon

¾ teaspoon ground star anise, plus more for garnish

½ teaspoon freshly grated nutmeg, plus more for garnish

5 cups (500 g) thick-cut old-fashioned oats (Bob's Red Mill is great)

1¼ cups (150 g) unsalted blanched Italian or Marcona almonds

1 cup (125 g) raw Sicilian pistachios

1 cup (75 g) unsweetened large flake coconut

1½ cups (165 g) unsulfured Turkish apricots, diced

1. Preheat the oven to 250°F (120°C) convection. Prepare a half sheet pan with a thin layer of olive oil to prevent sticking.

2. Place half of the orange zest in the bottom of a large mixing bowl.

3. Combine the orange juice, dates, olive oil, salt, and spices in a high-powered blender. Blend until smooth.

4. Transfer the date puree to the large bowl that contains the zest. Add the oats and stir to combine. Add the almonds, pistachios, and coconut and stir to combine.

5. Spread the mixture on the prepared half sheet pan. Bake for 30 minutes.

6. Stir the mixture, then return it to the oven and increase the temperature to 300°F (150°C). Bake for another 30 minutes.

7. Stir the mixture, then lower the heat back to 250°F (120°C) and bake for another 30 minutes. The mixture will have taken on a light golden color at this point.

8. Stir in the diced apricots, then increase the temperature again to 300°F (150°C) and bake for 20 to 30 minutes longer.

9. Remove from the oven and, while the mixture is still warm, sprinkle the remaining orange zest on top and add a few extra grates of nutmeg and star anise. Toss to combine and allow to cool completely.

10. Store in an airtight container for up to 3 weeks.

recipe continues . . .

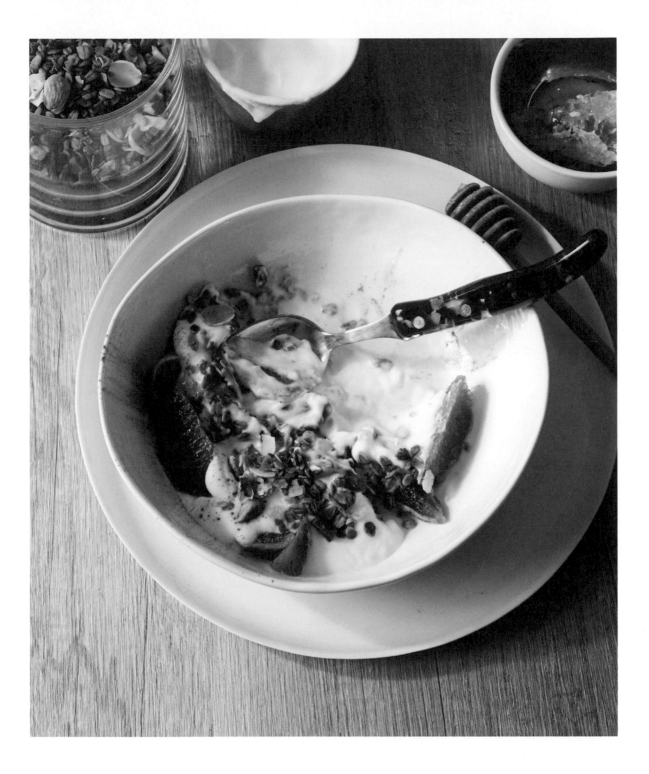

Fruit, wet, crunch: That's the ideal layering for granola bowls in my book. Place ¼ cup (about 140 g) whole, peeled segments of Ruby Red grapefruit with 2 quartered dried figs in the bottom of a bowl. Drape ¾ cup (180 g) goat's milk yogurt (for easier digestion) over the fruit and top with ¼ cup of Luxury Granola (page 22), a pinch of cinnamon, and raw honey. Serve with Designer Cashew Milk (page 13) on the side.

NOTES

Many homemade granola recipes require very short cooking times compared to this one, which is a *two-hour commitment*. But trust me; after much experience I am positive that the *slow and low* method is worth it and yields the best granola. You don't have to stir constantly, just every 30 minutes (or 15 if you are walking by the oven and feel the urge). Alternating the temperatures between 250° and 300°F (120° and 150°C) ensures evaporation and crisping without the burn of bitter granola.

Do not add the dried fruit until the last 30 minutes to prevent burned fruit. If you add them after cooking, the moisture left in the dried apricot always ends up making the granola soft.

Bronte pistachios are supergreen, superdelicious, imported from Sicily. You can replace with regular pistachios—they're just as delicious only slightly larger, a bit crunchier, and lacking that slight coconut essence that make the Bronte pistachio so unique. The almonds should be either blanched Italian almonds or Spanish Marcona. Both almonds are more buttery in flavor and texture than their California cousins.

SMOOTHIE BOWL

Can it really be . . . carrots in your smoothie bowl? Yes! This is a just-sweet-enough combination of bright orange to yellow juicy fruit and veggie powerhouses, without skimping at all on the alkalizing green shade we all know and love. Smoothie bowls tend to digest even better than their drinkable smoothie parents, because of a simple fact: You eat more slowly and mindfully with a spoon than you generally do with a straw. Cold smoothies do not light the digestive fire quite like a warm beverage; however, the slower and more mindfully you eat, the better you chew—yes, even a smoothie bowl—and the better you digest. In the cooler months, incorporate more warming spices (turmeric and cinnamon, for example) to keep your gut happy.

Makes 1 serving

BOWL

½ cup (60 g) frozen carrot,
  preblanched (see Notes)

⅓ cup (25 g) frozen spinach

¼ cup (30 g) frozen mango

¼ cup (30 g) frozen peach

½ teaspoon ground turmeric powder

¼ teaspoon ground Ceylon cinnamon

1 Proviotic

1 scant cup (225 ml) Designer
  Cashew Milk (page 13)

2 teaspoons (10 g) almond butter

½ teaspoon coconut oil

OPTIONAL TOPPINGS

1 tablespoon crushed raw or toasted
  hazelnuts

2 tablespoons wild blueberries

1 teaspoon bee pollen

1 tablespoon toasted unsweetened
  coconut flakes

1 tablespoon chia seeds

2 tablespoons Luxury Granola (page
  22)

1. Combine all the bowl ingredients in a high-powered blender.

2. Blend on high speed for 1½ minutes, starting on low speed and using a spatula or the blender plunger to move the smoothie around.

3. Gradually adjust the blender speed, ending on high speed to fully puree the mixture, about 1 minute in total. Use a spatula to scrape into a bowl.

4. Add toppings as desired.

NOTES

The toppings are up to your own imagination. Think of a balance of additional flavor, fat, and vitamins, with bee pollen containing complex carbohydrates along with a complex amino acid and mineral profile (the building blocks of muscle); blueberries, rich in antioxidants; chia seeds for extra protein and fiber; hazelnuts for protein, fiber, and flavor; and coconut for antimicrobial fat and fiber.

Carrots do not steam very well, so better to blanch them (briefly submerge) in boiling water for 5 minutes, or until soft. Allow the carrots to cool before placing in the freezer for your smoothie prep.

BLANK CANVAS PORRIDGE

It may sound completely absurd and not applicable to flake and grind your own oats. You can buy them just about anywhere for practically nothing—why would you complicate something so basic? But freshly ground oats were one of the things that changed my eating life forever, so I decided I must recruit every reader to this insane-but-worth-it step.

Oatmeal porridge is my ultimate blank canvas. The toppings are an extension of the atmosphere I want to create for myself. When the groats are freshly cracked and prepared, they develop a full-bodied aroma and taste that just calls out to be topped with freshly halved apricots and a dollop of goat's milk yogurt. Elegance and simplicity.

Oats contain complex carbohydrates, meaning they digest more slowly than a refined or processed carbohydrate, keeping your insulin (blood sugar) levels stable. Carbohydrates are not bad! Fear not, for they are sources of energy. When you find yourself asking, "Should I eat carbs?" just think: *How hungry am I? What is my activity level going to be today?* Everyone's carbohydrate needs differ, so it is important as you discover your Clean Enough to tune in to how food, including oatmeal, makes you feel and perform.

Makes 2 servings

2¾ cups (660 ml) filtered water

1 cup (100 g) flaked oat groats (about ⅔ cup/65 g unflaked; see Notes) or thick-cut rolled oats (Bob's Red Mill is a great variety)

¼ teaspoon scraped vanilla bean seeds

Pinch of Himalayan pink salt

OPTIONAL TOPPINGS (USE YOUR IMAGINATION!)

European Holiday: goat's milk yogurt + fresh apricot halves + freshly grated nutmeg

Creamsicle: Designer Cashew Milk (page 13) + unsweetened coconut flakes + fresh passion fruit + grated orange zest

Honey Nut: sliced banana + raw honey + nut butter + ground Ceylon cinnamon

Savory: raw hemp seeds + Hazelnut Arugula (page 54) + seared mushrooms (from Longevity Mushroom Toast, page 39)

1. Bring the water to a simmer in a medium saucepan over medium-high and whisk in the oats, vanilla bean seeds, and salt.

2. Simmer for 10 minutes, whisking, until the oats are tender and the water is absorbed.

3. Divide the porridge between two bowls.

4. While the porridge is hot, top as preferred.

NOTE

You can purchase a hand-cranked oat flaker or KitchenAid oat flaker attachment from Amazon. This is well worth the investment. While I prefer to grind right before I prepare the oats, similar to freshly ground coffee, you can always grind or flake a few batches of oat groats for your week ahead. I have made my granola, porridge, and overnight oats from both freshly flaked and purchased thick-cut rolled oats.

RUNNY EGG BOWL

In my early pastry days, I do not think I ever ate real food, instead subsisting off broken cookies and fruit remnants. Runny eggs, in their simplicity and swift execution, was what I started with when I began to teach myself to eat properly, with intention and pause, subsequently normalizing my life almost immediately. With so much protein, eggs are a versatile energy source, certainly sugar-free, and satiate without having to consume a lot of volume of food. I prefer my eggs to be runny—in this case, soft-boiled, poached, or sunny-side up—as the yolks' nutrients are easier to process when not hard-cooked. Personally, I prefer to not eat eggs *every day*, instead making them a part of my diet *weekly*.

Makes 2 servings

SOFT-BOILED EGGS

4 pasture-raised eggs

1. Place the eggs in small, heavy-bottomed saucepan and add room-temperature water to cover.

2. Place the pan over high heat and as soon as the water comes to a boil, turn off the heat, immediately setting a 5-minute timer. Prepare a small bowl of ice and water; set aside.

3. When the timer goes off, place the eggs in the ice water to stop the cooking.

4. Peel the cooled eggs and rewarm by placing in warm water before serving.

....

POACHED EGGS

2 tablespoons white vinegar

2 teaspoons fine sea salt

4 pasture-raised eggs

1. Bring a small, heavy-bottomed saucepan of water to a boil.

2. Lower the heat to a simmer and add the vinegar and salt.

3. Swirl the water and gently crack one egg in.

4. Turn off the heat and place a lid on the pot. Allow the egg to poach for 4 minutes.

5. Remove the poached egg with a slotted spoon and drain on a paper tower until ready to serve. Repeat to poach the remaining three eggs, one at a time.

SUNNY-SIDE-UP EGGS

4 pasture-raised eggs

1 teaspoon extra virgin olive oil

1. Heat a small nonstick skillet or seasoned cast-iron skillet over medium heat.

2. Add ¼ teaspoon of the olive oil and crack one egg into the skillet.

3. Place a plate or pot lid on top of the skillet to allow the heat to circulate, cooking the white evenly.

4. Remove the egg when the white is cooked and the yolk is beautifully set yet still runny. Repeat to cook the other three eggs, one at a time.

....

EGG BOWL

2 teaspoons extra virgin olive oil

2 cups (300 g) cherry tomatoes

1½ cups (60 g) lacinto kale, stemmed and roughly chopped into 1-inch (2.5 cm) ribbons

Heavy pinch of freshly ground black pepper

Heavy pinch of Himalayan pink salt

Pinch of crushed red pepper flakes

½ avocado, peeled, pitted, and chopped into ½-inch (13 mm) pieces

4 runny eggs: poached, soft-boiled, or sunny-side up (pages 27–28)

3 tablespoons Tahini Dressing, below

Super Seed Blend (page 108), optional

1. Heat the olive oil in a cast-iron skillet over medium-high heat. Add the tomatoes and allow them to sear until they begin to burst.

2. Add the chopped kale to the skillet after the tomatoes begin to blister, then season with black pepper, salt, and red pepper flakes. Sauté for 2 minutes to wilt the kale.

3. Once the kale is wilted, turn off the heat and add the chopped avocado.

4. Divide the vegetable mixture between two bowls and top each bowl with two runny eggs of your choice.

5. Drizzle the eggs and vegetables with Tahini Dressing and add Super Seed Blend to taste to season.

TAHINI DRESSING

Makes 1 scant cup (225 ml)

2 tablespoons (30 g) tahini paste

½ teaspoons sumac

½ teaspoons za'atar

¼ teaspoon freshly ground black pepper

¼ teaspoon grated lemon zest

¼ teaspoon Himalayan pink salt

2 tablespoons filtered water

1 tablespoons fresh lemon juice

Whisk together all the ingredients in a medium bowl. Use immediately.

OVERNIGHT OATS

Muesli—read: overnight oats—has seen a resurgence with the notion of their being both grab-and-go-able *and* homemade (usually in a mason jar to boot) on busy mornings. The secret to these oats is to keep it light with the addition of apple cider instead of using only nut milk for your soaking liquid. A heavy dusting of cinnamon and freshly sliced pears taste amazing with a hearty scoop of soaked oats. No need to warm; enjoy cool or at room temperature. This is a nutrient- and energy-dense dish full of whole foods. Even carrots! They provide a sweet flavor and pair well with the apples. Eat this as a premade breakfast, helping you reach for a healthy choice, or have a smaller portion as a snack in the midafternoon if you are hungry and low energy.

Makes 4 servings

1 cup (240 ml) Designer Cashew Milk (page 13), plus more to serve

½ cup (120 ml) unfiltered apple cider

½ teaspoon coconut oil

¼ teaspoon ground cardamom

½ Granny Smith apple, grated with peel on (3½ ounces/100 g)

1 cup (100 g) thick-cut old-fashioned oats (I prefer Bob's Red Mill)

⅓ cup (50 g) unsulfured Turkish apricots, diced

¼ cup (30 g) peeled and grated carrot

¼ cup (15 g) unsweetened large flake coconut

2 tablespoons raw chopped walnuts

1 tablespoon (10 g) chia seeds

½ teaspoon ground Ceylon cinnamon, plus more to serve

1 cup (160 g) sliced pear or other fresh fruit

1. Whisk together the cashew milk, apple cider, coconut oil, and cardamom in a large bowl.

2. Stir in the grated apple, oats, apricots, carrot, coconut flakes, walnuts, and chia seeds.

3. Transfer to an airtight container, dusting the top of the mixture heavily with cinnamon to create a distinct layer.

4. Place in the refrigerator for 4 hours or overnight.

5. To serve, place ½ cup (125 g) soaked oats in a bowl and top with additional cinnamon. Add additional cashew milk to thin, if desired, and top with ¼ cup (40 g) sliced pear.

SOFT SCRAMBLED EGGS WITH RADISHES

A bowl of soft scrambled eggs with a bit of chive, a piece of hearty whole grain black bread, and some fresh radishes. What a lovely morning!

Cooking your eggs until they are just softly scrambled is the secret. By doing this and not whipping your eggs, you create a naturally creamy and dense egg without the addition of butter, milk, or cream. Seasoning the eggs after they cook also prevents the proteins in the eggs from becoming too firm, so be sure to hold the salt until then.

Black bread, or dark rye, creates a rich and creamy caramel flavor with a little schmear of goat butter and blue poppy seeds. Spicy radishes complement the soft eggs and hearty toast. This complete meal contains energizing whole grains; whole protein; satiating fats found in the egg yolks, olive oil, and goat's butter; bitter vegetables that act as a great digestive aid; and mineral-rich blue poppy seeds.

Makes 2 servings

2 slices black bread
  (dark buckwheat rye)

4 large pasture-raised eggs

1 teaspoon minced fresh chives

½ teaspoon extra virgin olive oil

Maldon sea salt flakes

Freshly ground black pepper

1 teaspoon goat's milk butter

1 cup (100 g) quartered radishes

1 teaspoon blue poppy seeds

2 lemon wedges (⅛ lemon)

1. Toast the bread, slice each piece in half, and allow to cool slightly (I prefer my toast with not totally melted butter, so the cooling is essential).

2. Meanwhile, gently whisk the eggs in a small bowl. Add the minced chives and stir to just combine. Do not overwhip the eggs at this point.

3. Heat the olive oil in a small nonstick or cast-iron skillet over medium-low heat. Add the eggs and immediately begin scraping them toward the center, using a heatproof rubber spatula.

4. Cook the eggs until just scrambled, remove from the heat, and season with salt and pepper to taste. Divide between two small bowls.

5. While the eggs are cooking, melt ½ teaspoon of the goat butter in a small saucepan. Add the quartered radishes and toss to just glaze without cooking. Season with a hearty pinch of salt and half of the poppy seeds.

6. Place the radishes alongside the scrambled eggs in the bowls.

7. Schmear the remaining goat's milk butter on each halved piece of toast (¼ teaspoon per slice of bread), finishing with a sprinkle of poppy seeds.

8. Serve the toast perched on the edge of each bowl of eggs along with a wedge of lemon.

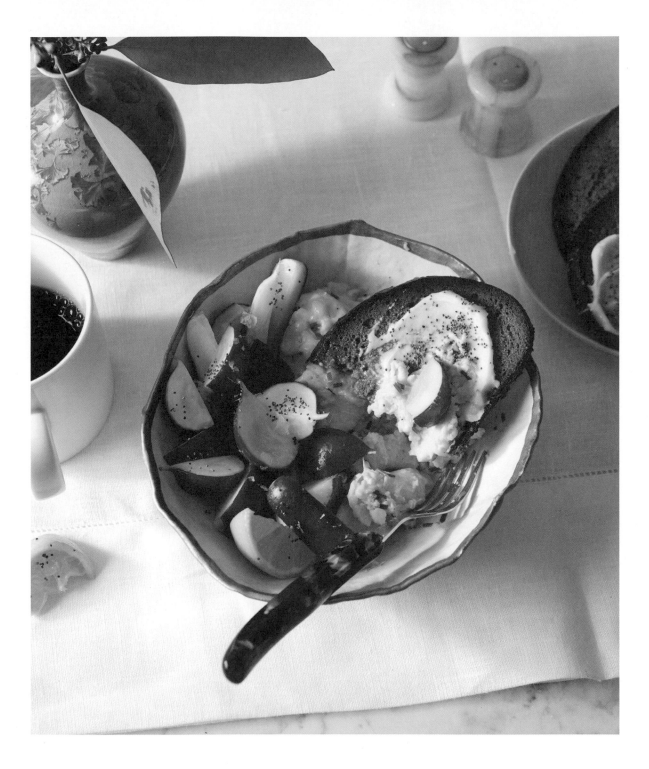

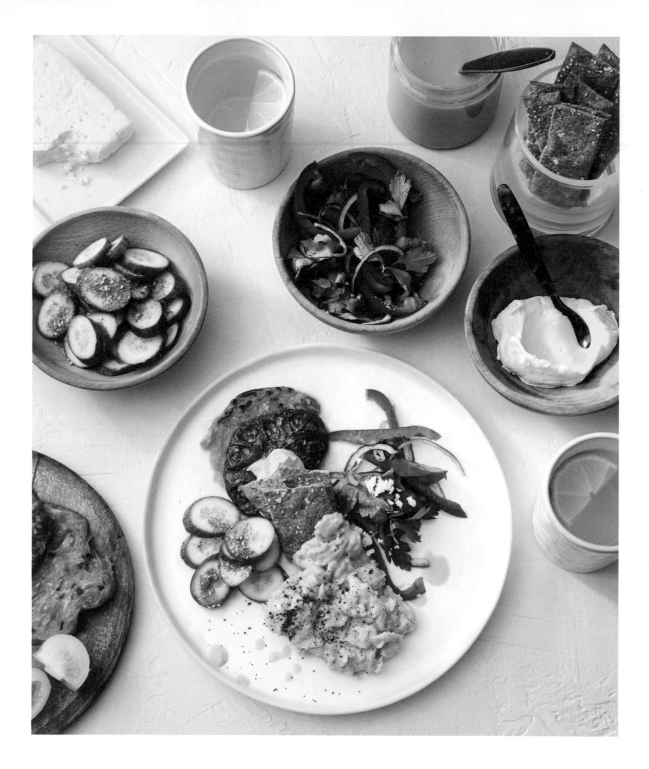

ISRAELI BREAKFAST

Israel was at the tail end of my first around-the-world tour. I had spent a month on the road with my boss, Sam, and we had shared many meals and many (many) bread baskets, along with a lot of time sitting on an airplane. He was exasperated with the tightening of his trousers, and by the time we reached Israel, we had boycotted any more baked goods. Israel was a great way to reset our digestion and food choices, mainly with the fresh spread known as Israeli breakfast. While this traditionally is served with lavash bread, lavash is not the centerpiece of the meal. Rather, you will find a delicious meze of organic eggs, probiotic-rich yogurt, light and flavorful feta, cleansing herb salads, juicy tomatoes, such antioxidant herbs as sumac, and nutritious tahini. Israeli breakfast is Clean Enough in its purest essence. I will forever fondly remember those breakfasts—on top of all of the philosophical conversations about life, love, food, art, and culture we had while sharing them. This recipe is excellent for a group brunch, but it can easily be made smaller when your body is craving energy and vitamins (aka, healthy indulgence).

Makes 4 servings

8 large pasture-raised eggs

¼ cup (60 g) tahini paste

4 slices heirloom tomato, each ½ inch (13 mm) thick

2½ teaspoons extra virgin olive oil

4 Persian cucumbers (7 ounces/ 200 g)

1 teaspoon za'atar

½ cup (80 g) diced red onion

1 large red bell pepper, seeded and sliced thin

1 cup (60 g) fresh parsley leaves

1 teaspoon ground cumin

½ teaspoon grated lemon zest

¼ teaspoon Himalayan pink salt

¼ teaspoon freshly ground black pepper

½ cup (115 g) Labne (page 109)

½ teaspoon sumac

Super Seed Blend (page 108), optional

Flatbread or whole grain crackers for serving

1. Crack the eggs into a bowl and add the tahini. Using an immersion stick blender, blend the mixture together.

2. Separately, turn on the oven broiler. Place the tomato slices on a small sheet pan directly under the broiler and broil for 5 minutes.

3. Meanwhile, heat ½ teaspoon of the olive oil in a nonstick skillet over high heat and add the egg mixture. Scrape the eggs toward the center of the pan, using a heatproof rubber spatula. Continue to drag the eggs into the center to cook quickly and remove from the heat before the eggs seem "done," as they will continue to cook away from the heat.

4. Slice the Persian cucumber and toss with the za'atar. Place in a small serving bowl.

5. Soak the red onion in cold water for 10 minutes. Drain, then combine with the remaining 2 teaspoons olive oil, the bell pepper, parsley, cumin, lemon zest, salt, and black pepper. Place in a small serving bowl.

6. To serve, place one broiled tomato slice in the bottom of each of your individual bowls with 1 tablespoon of Labne on top.

7. Dividing equally among the four bowls, portion the scrambled eggs directly on top of the melty, broiled tomato.

8. Sprinkle the eggs with the sumac and Super Seed Blend, if using. Serve with the herbed onion salad, cucumbers, additional Labne and tahini, and flatbread.

GREEN FAVA BAKED EGGS

Shakshuka: soft, bubbling tomato sauce swirled with pureed fava, Rose Harissa (page 117), and eggs. Flavor forward without any excess and perfect for sharing. The tomato sauce creates a base to nestle in organic eggs, allowing them to cook slowly, suspended in warming spices, vibrant vegetables, the heart-healthy beans, and a special Tunisian hot sauce. This is food of the magical healing variety. Serve with crusty bread for a weekend brunch or alternatively as a comforting breakfast-for-dinner scenario.

Makes 4 servings

FAVA BEAN PUREE (SEE NOTES)

2 cups (300 g) dried peeled fava beans

1 tablespoon extra virgin olive oil

2 teaspoons fresh oregano leaves

½ teaspoon grated lemon zest

1 teaspoon fresh lemon juice

1 teaspoon Himalayan pink salt

½ teaspoon ground turmeric

¼ teaspoon black pepper

BAKED EGGS IN SAUCE

1 tablespoon extra virgin olive oil

1 small white or yellow onion, sliced
  thinly (½ cup/80 g)

1 to 2 garlic cloves, sliced

½ teaspoon ground cumin

½ teaspoon smoked paprika

2 cups (450 g) crushed tomatoes

½ cup (120 ml) filtered water

1 teaspoon Himalayan pink salt

1 teaspoon freshly ground black pepper

2 ounces (55 g) goat's milk feta

4 large pasture-raised eggs

½ cup (115 g) Rose Harissa (page 117)

½ teaspoon sumac

1. To make the beans: Rinse the dried favas and place in a medium pot. Cover with filtered water extending 2 inches (5 cm) above the layer of beans in the pot. Bring to a boil over high heat, then turn off the heat and allow the beans to sit, covered, for 1 hour.

2. Strain the beans and place back in the pot, covering with fresh water to 5 inches (12.5 cm) above the layer of beans. Bring the beans to a boil and allow to simmer for 1 hour, or until tender. Allow the beans to cool in the cooking liquid. (Don't discard that liquid!)

3. To make the eggs: Heat the olive oil in a small to medium sauté pan or cast-iron skillet over medium-low heat and add the onion and garlic. Sauté without burning for 10 minutes. Add the cumin and paprika and stir to coat the onion mixture with the spices.

4. Add the tomatoes, water, salt, and pepper. Cover and simmer over low heat for 20 minutes to reduce the tomatoes.

5. Meanwhile, prepare the puree: Strain the beans, reserving ½ cup (120 ml) of the bean cooking liquid. Combine 1 cup (170 g) of the beans, the reserved cooking liquid, olive oil, oregano, lemon zest and juice, salt, and turmeric in a high-powered blender. Blend to make a smooth puree.

6. Once the tomato sauce has simmered, turn off the heat and taste for seasoning. Add additional salt and pepper, if desired.

7. Place dollops of fava puree and Rose Harissa on top of the tomato sauce. Very lightly, swirl the fava puree and harissa into the sauce, leaving a clear delineation between the three ingredients. Sprinkle with the crumbled feta.

recipe continues . . .

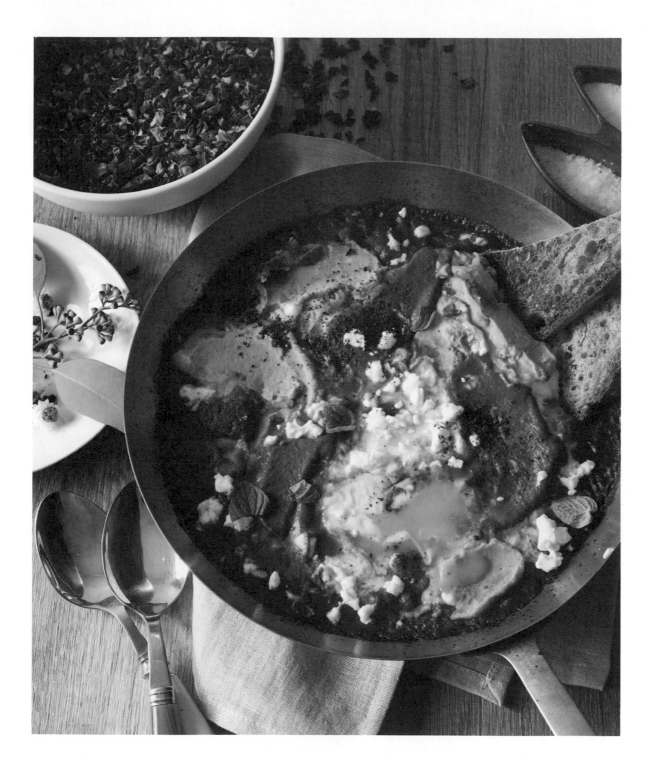

8. Using a spoon, make four nests in the tomato sauce mixture and carefully crack an egg into each hole. Cover the pan and continue to cook the sauce over low heat, allowing the egg whites to cook with the yolks remaining runny, about 5 minutes.

9. Remove the pan from the heat and sprinkle with sumac before serving directly from the pan with crusty bread.

NOTES

You will have leftover cooked fava beans (the recipe makes around 4 cups/680 g cooked beans). Use these beans in salads or make an extra batch or two of fava bean puree to have on hand as a dip or snack with crackers or crudités, or as a salad topper for extra protein.

TOPPED TOAST

There's a reason that we turn to toast in the mornings: It is unbelievably grounding. Less of a commitment than a full sandwich, but still hearty enough and an excellent energy source. A topped toast really gets you to stop, even for a moment. Whether served as a simple breakfast, a light lunch, a casual dinner, or alongside other prepared vegetables, salads, soups, or dessert, toast deserves your respect. I like to make toasts (not finger sandwiches, mind you) as a little surprise for guests when they come over. Even if they think they want an elaborate meal, show them a crispy piece of whole grain miche sourdough toast with a few perfect schmears of mashed peas and they may melt. With bread, the type of vehicle, make, and model, is entirely up to you. To keep it Clean Enough, I encourage finding whole grain breads that you like from bakers who mill their own flour or source high-quality milled grains for their loaves. Why? Fresh cracked grains contain the most nutrients and the most flavor bang for your buck; ensure that the whole grain is used rather than processed and refined flours. Sourdough, a naturally fermented and leavened product, is a great choice for digestive health, with heartier six-grain breads offering nutrient density. When in doubt, just ask or read the label.

Once you find a few types of bread—mainly a dark rye, multigrain, and sourdough that you love—you can keep those as back-pocket staples in your freezer for toast in a pinch, leaving room to explore new varieties as you come across them. Please patronize your local baker here, just like your local farmer. Get to know them and their practices, as their craft is an art. These experts possess the kind of skills and Midas touch you can safely rely on as a resource to support your Clean Enough journey.

AVOCADO GUACAMOLE TOAST

This is how I like my guacamole, which is why I like my toast to be merely a vehicle for this fresh and flavorful mash. Avocado is an excellent postworkout recovery meal full of monounsaturated fat, specifically oleonic acid, providing anti-inflammatory benefits as well as a balanced nervous system, thanks to the high level of vitamin E. Avocado toast and fitness classes seem to go hand in hand, a trend that need not go away as moving and nourishing your body well are two key components to feeling Enough.

Makes 4 servings

2 organic avocados

4 teaspoons extra virgin olive oil

4 slices whole grain miche or whole grain sourdough bread, each 1 inch (2.5 cm) thick

1 teaspoon Himalayan pink salt

1 teaspoon freshly ground black pepper

¼ cup (30 g) thinly sliced radish (paper thin)

1 teaspoon ground cumin

1 teaspoon red pepper flakes

4 teaspoons minced red onion

4 teaspoons crumbled goat's milk feta (20 g)

2 tablespoons pumpkin seeds, toasted and lightly salted

2 tablespoons fresh cilantro leaves

4 lime or lemon wedges (⅛ lime or lemon)

1. Heat a small nonstick or cast-iron grill pan over high heat.

2. Cut the avocados in half, discard the pits, and rub each cut half with a few drops of the olive oil. Place the halved avocados (skin on), flesh side down, on the pan. Grill for 30 seconds until just charred, then set aside.

3. Toast the bread slices underneath the broiler in an oven or in a toaster oven until deep golden. Drizzle the toasted bread with the remaining olive oil and sprinkle with a heavy pinch of the salt and black pepper.

4. Using a paring knife, slice each avocado half lengthwise in the skin into about eight slices each. Using a spoon, scoop the flesh from each avocado half onto each slice of toast, mashing slightly.

5. Wedge slices of radish into the mashed avocado. Season the avocado with the remaining salt and black pepper and the cumin and red pepper flakes.

6. Sprinkle each toast with red onion, crumbled feta, pumpkin seeds, and fresh cilantro. Place a citrus wedge at the edge of each toast.

VARIATION

Make this a flavorful and powerful gut-friendly toast full of probiotics by adding a schmear of Miso Dressing (page 108) on top of the toasted bread prior to adding the avocado. Top with Kraut (page 112).

LONGEVITY MUSHROOM TOAST

This toast calls for a fork and a steak knife, a courtyard at dusk, and glass of red. All ingredients of a long and well-lived life. Pan-seared mineral-rich mushrooms sit atop deeply toasted whole grain sourdough, with the juices soaking straight into the bread. Mushrooms come in many varieties, all with their own unique flavor profile and active health- and energy-supporting compounds—all the more reason to use a combination when preparing this toast. Did I mention that just one small portion of mushrooms—yes, a single mushroom a day—has been shown to block tumor growth and decrease the risk of some cancers by 60 percent? The white button mushroom is humble no more. Paired with pungent and equally as hearty thyme with its own host of benefits, including being a strong diuretic, this flavorful toast proves that clean food can be craveable.

Makes 2 generous servings or 4 side servings

1 tablespoon + 1 teaspoon extra virgin olive oil

1 shallot, sliced paper thin

½ teaspoon grated garlic

4 cups (300 g) mixed mushrooms (e.g., baby portobello, hen of the woods, white button, shiitake)

1 tablespoon + 1 teaspoon fresh thyme leaves

1 teaspoon freshly ground black pepper, plus a pinch for sprinkling

½ teaspoon Himalayan pink salt, plus a pinch for sprinkling

⅔ cup (160 ml) organic unsalted vegetable stock

1 teaspoon fresh lemon juice

2 slices miche or other whole grain sourdough bread, each 1 inch (2.5 cm) thick

4 teaspoons Labne (page 109)

2 tablespoons (10 g) thinly grated aged Manchego or any other aged hard sheep's milk cheese

1. Wash dirt from mushrooms. If they're large, cut into smaller (1½ inch/4 cm) chunks.

2. Heat a cast-iron skillet on medium heat. Heat 1 tablespoon of the olive oil and add the shallot and garlic. Sauté for 1 minute and then add the mushrooms, thyme, pepper, and salt. Sauté over medium-high heat for about 4 minutes, or until the mushrooms are tender and seared.

3. Add the vegetable stock and lemon juice to deglaze the pan, scraping up any browned bits that are stuck to the bottom. Simmer for 3 to 4 more minutes.

4. Meanwhile, place the sourdough bread slices under the broiler, in a toaster oven, or on a grill to toast until deep golden.

5. Drizzle the hot toast with the remaining teaspoon of olive oil and season with a pinch each of salt and pepper. Schmear each piece of toast with Labne.

6. Place the toasts on individual serving plates or on a platter and top with the seared mushrooms, scraping out every morsel to soak into the toast. Top with shavings of Manchego.

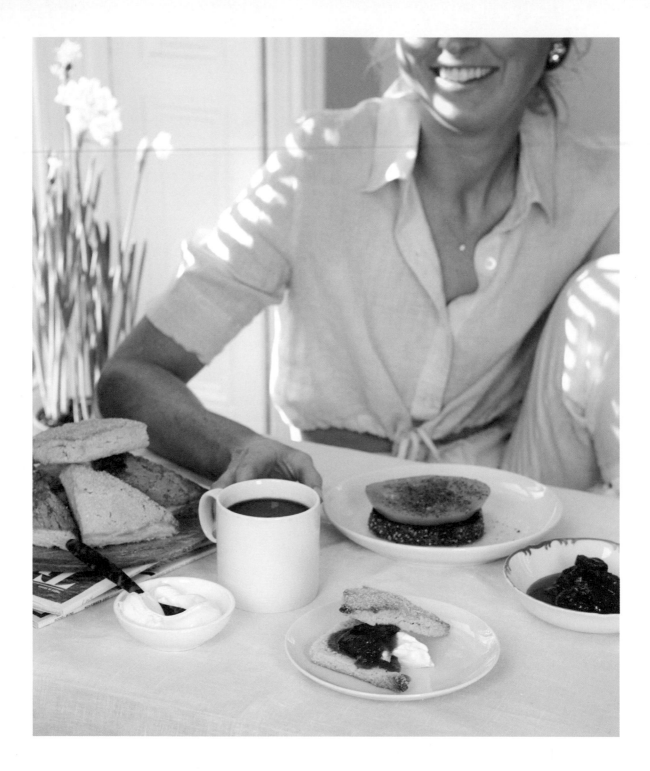

ACK TOMATO TOAST

Nantucket (ACK) is one of my favorite places on Earth; I just feel something there. I am happy. Maybe it's baked into the island's on-site bakery, the one that makes the absolute best beach sandwiches on its signature six-grain bread that I bring home with me to keep in the freezer for when beach season has passed, making it the ultimate base to this simple toast. Be a curious consumer, as good whole grain bread can be junk food in disguise. Read the ingredients label, as dough softener, added sugar, and preservatives are decidedly not Clean Enough. Something Natural, both the name of the bakery and the ingredients in its whole grain bread, brings integrity to the simplicity of eating clean food. Simple food encourages you to eat with the seasons and this toast does just that, with tomatoes—at their peak August through September—flowing with your body's natural rhythm.

Makes 4 servings

4 slices six-grain or other whole grain multigrain bread, each ½ inch (13 mm) thick

2 teaspoons goat's milk butter

½ teaspoon Himalayan pink salt

4 slices large heirloom tomatoes (160 g), each ½ inch (13 mm) thick

1 teaspoon freshly ground black pepper

1. Toast the bread slices under a broiler or in a toaster oven until deep golden.

2. Spread a thin layer of goat's butter on the warm toast and sprinkle salt on top of the butter.

3. Place the tomato slices on top and finish with loads of freshly ground black pepper.

NOTES

My ultimate summer tomatoes come from Bartlett's Farm on Nantucket. I also love an heirloom variety called Hawaiian gold, which is bright, juicy, and sweet. Check out the local section of your grocery store or the farmer's market for large, juicy heirloom varieties.

I prefer to salt my bread and then grind pepper directly onto the tomato. As ripe tomatoes contain a lot of juice, salting directly will merely draw out more juice unnecessarily.

Adding a runny egg (pages 27–28) makes this more of a complete meal rather than a lighter breakfast or snack.

Serve this alongside soup, such as Fermented Garlic and Squash Soup (page 99) as well as salad, such as the Honeycrisp Whole Grain and Pecorino salad (page 53).

PIRBRIGHT PEA AND MINT TOAST

I love bright green peas, fresh off the vine in spring, petite nutrient-rich powerhouses full of naturally sweet flavor. There is something so deeply satisfying about taking the simple peas one step further with a mash, a British vegetable staple. The addition of fresh mint not only adds a layer a flavor sans additional salt and fat, it aids in the digestion of this nurturing toast topper. I remember fondly afternoon teas when I was fifteen, prepared at Older Lodge, an old friend's house in Pirbright, Surrey. I could be found either trying to catch a moment with my friend's older brother, whom I had the biggest crush on, or in the kitchen, floating in and out of jet lag. This historic manor had an old-school gas stove called an AGA, where you would place your bread between two wire screens before inserting into the hinged door to brown. Out would come toast, accompanied by a table spread that included a pot of jam, a crock of butter, tea, and a bowl of warm peas from the night prior.

Makes 3 servings

1 cup (150 g) shelled fresh peas (or frozen)

1½ teaspoons unsalted goat's milk butter

1 shallot, sliced paper thin

1 teaspoon unsalted vegetable stock or filtered water

1½ tablespoons chopped fresh mint leaves

2 teaspoons (5 g) grated aged Parmesan

1 teaspoon fresh lemon juice

⅛ teaspoon Himalayan pink salt

Pinch of freshly ground black pepper

3 thin slices dark rye or whole grain sourdough bread, each about 1 cm thick

1. Bring 3 cups (720 ml) water to a boil in a small saucepan. Add the peas and cook for 30 seconds. Drain immediately and set aside.

2. Heat 1 teaspoon of the butter in the saucepan just used for the peas and add the shallot. Sweat the shallot over medium-low heat for 5 minutes, or until translucent. Add water or vegetable stock.

3. Add the peas back to the saucepan and stir to warm and combine.

4. Transfer the peas mixture to a food processor along with 1 tablespoon of the mint leaves. Season with 1 teaspoon of the Parmesan, the lemon juice, salt, and pepper. Pulse until smooth.

5. Toast the bread slices underneath the broiler or in a toaster oven until light golden.

6. Spread a scant amount (½ teaspoon) of the remaining goat's butter on each toast followed by 2 heaping tablespoons of pea mash.

7. Spread the mash on each toast with the back of a spoon and sprinkle with the remaining teaspoon of grated Parmesan.

NOTES

To make this a meal, place the toast in the bottom of a bowl and pile the Kale and Preserved Lemon Caesar Salad (page 48) or Radish Peas Parmesan Salad (page 52) on top with the addition of an optional runny egg (pages 27–28).

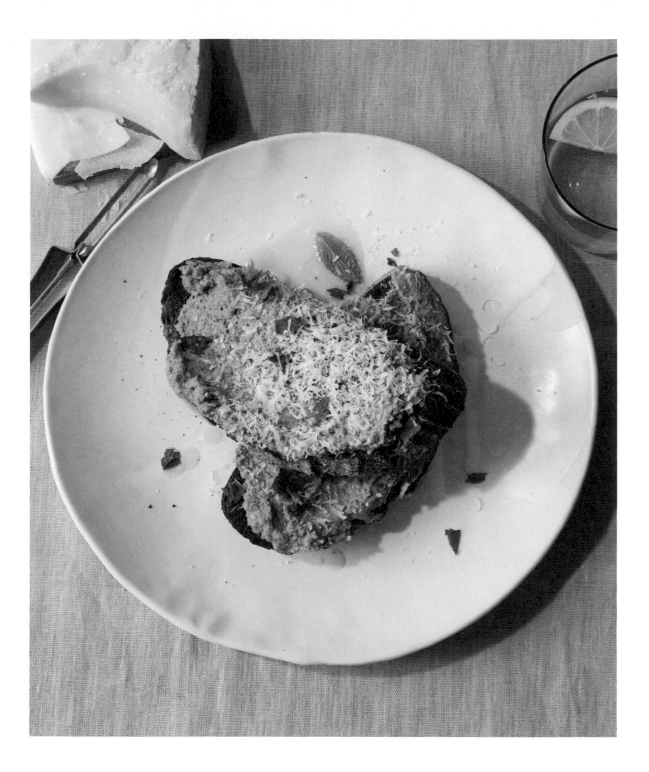

TOPPED TOAST

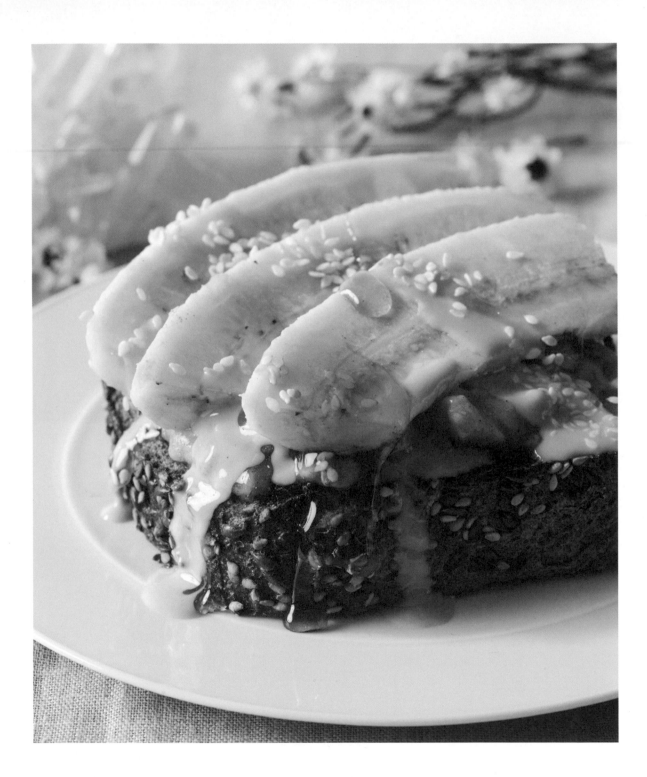

TAHINI BANANA BEE TOAST

Y ou may take the humble banana for granted until you take a bite of this toast, which is basically a new form of food-texture healing. Mashed jellylike banana, sticky tahini paste, sesame seeds wrapped up in tongue-to-the-roof-of-your-mouth raw honey, all atop crispy whole grain bread. This toast is straight clean energy, fulfilling all three of your macronutrient needs: fat, protein, and carbs. For days that are activity heavy and in need of simple, easy-to-digest fuel. The same goes for a hungry afternoon feeling, for something borderline dessert when you have already had enough.

Makes 2 servings

2 slices six-grain or other whole grain
   multigrain bread, each ½ inch
   (13 mm) thick

2 organic bananas

½ teaspoon ground Ceylon cinnamon,
   plus more for sprinkling

2 tablespoons tahini paste

2 teaspoons raw honey

2 teaspoon white sesame seeds

1. Toast the whole grain bread slices underneath a broiler or in a toaster oven until very golden.

2. In a small bowl, mash one banana with the cinnamon, using a fork. Divide between the two toasts, spreading evenly.

3. Drizzle the toasts with the tahini paste.

4. Slice the second banana in half lengthwise and then into thirds. Divide the banana slices between both toasts and drizzle with the honey.

5. Sprinkle generously with the sesame seeds and additional cinnamon.

NOTES

In a single 2-tablespoon (28 g) serving, sesame seeds contribute protein along with a considerable amount of vitamins and minerals, including calcium, essential for bone health, and magnesium, which helps stabilize blood sugar and acts as a mood booster.

Potassium-rich bananas, another nutrient essential for bone health, also contain magnesium.

GREENS
(SALAD, MOSTLY RAW)

Greens are one of the few universal recommendations to add more of to your diet to improve health outcomes and digestion and create a more alkaline and balanced state of being. They are a great place to start when coaching yourself to add clean foods, rather than focusing on eliminating all the foods that you have deemed bad.

Greens is a loose term in this section, referring to (mostly) raw salads, with a variety of greens, bitter lettuces, other vegetables, and a wide range of simple yet flavorful dressings to match. Each dish in this section can act as a great side, a simple meal, or the base to a bowl, with grains as a topping rather than the main event. Color is important here: Not only do you eat with your eyes, but color indicates vitamins, which all serve to support optimum cell function—a combination of happiness and science in a salad.

With all of this talk about raw vegetables, it is important to reference the Dirty Dozen. The Environmental Working Group (EWG) issues this list of fruits and vegetables that are best purchased organic.

DIRTY DOZEN

Strawberries	Pears	Bell Peppers
Spinach	Cherries	Potatoes
Nectarines	Grapes	Hot Peppers
Apples	Celery	
Peaches	Tomatoes	

CLEAN 15

Sweet Corn	Sweet Peas	Honeydew Melon
Avocado	Papaya	Kiwi
Pineapple	Asparagus	Cantaloupe
Cabbage	Mangoes	Cauliflower
Onions	Eggplant	Grapefruit

2017 EWG Dirty Dozen and Clean 15 List. Visit ewg.org

LITTLE BLACK DRESSED GREENS

I love referring to this version of my back-pocket staple as simply "greens," never "salad." Greens are one of the few foods that you can eat with slight abandon, given their low calories and high water content. When I was first in New York, I had an odd schedule, weekends during the week and dinners always late and hurried. I often made a big bowl of this salad in a pinch, bringing me a sense of grounding and some nutrients after being on my feet all day grazing on ciabatta doughnuts that didn't make it to the plate. The dressing is unbelievably simple, yet every time I make it I am always asked, without fail, "What is in this dressing?" The key is grating your fresh garlic directly into the bottom of the bowl and using (clean) hands to slosh around the fresh lemon juice and quality extra virgin olive oil before tossing in the leaves. I may have had zero balance in my life in my early twenties, but I am grateful for these greens that are still to this day my favorite.

Makes 6 servings

1 garlic clove, peeled

1 teaspoon freshly ground black pepper

½ teaspoon Himalayan pink salt

Juice of ½ lemon

3 tablespoons extra virgin olive oil

About 5½ ounces (3 cups/160 g) mixed mesclun greens

About 4 ounces (2 cups/110 g) torn radicchio leaves

About 3 ounces (4 cups/80 g) baby arugula

Super Seed Blend (page 108), optional

1. Grate the raw garlic directly into a large salad bowl.

2. Add the pepper and salt and mash with your (clean) fingers or the back of a soupspoon.

3. Add the lemon juice and stir. Drizzle in the olive oil and combine well. In small batches, add all the greens and toss lightly with your hands.

4. Add the Super Seed Blend, if using, to season, and serve immediately.

NOTES

It is important to use an extra virgin olive oil that you love, as it is not only a great fat that helps your body absorb the vitamins in the leafy greens, but also a great opportunity to add a distinctive favor.

Use this recipe as a lighter base for a nourishing grain bowl, using grains or legumes as a topping (such as the Miso Brown Rice, page 82), along with Charred Pumpkin Seed Broccolini (page 72), Blistered Miso Sweet Potatoes (page 83), and Kraut (page 112) for digestion.

KALE AND PRESERVED LEMON CAESAR

Kale, a fiber-rich cruciferous vegetable, is full of a host of minerals, including iron and calcium, essential for cell growth, bone density, and a healthy metabolism. Raw, dry curly kale makes me sad inside. Why would you ever force someone to partake in something like that when a little massage or steam goes such a long way, breaking down the cellulose in the hearty green for a more pleasant dining experience? This can be achieved as easily as adding a squeeze of lemon and a bit of muscle; in this case, I prefer to massage the kale with an ultraflavorful dressing full of lemon, both preserved and fresh. This salad always makes an appearance at a Thanksgiving dinner that I cohost annually with my brother, Matt, adding a little dimension to the standard fare.

Makes 3 servings

PRESERVED LEMON CAESAR DRESSING

1½ ounces (35 g) preserved lemon rind, seeds removed (¼ lemon)

¼ cup (30 g) raw cashews

1 tablespoon pine nuts

1 garlic clove, peeled

1½ teaspoons freshly ground black pepper

¾ teaspoon Himalayan pink salt

½ teaspoon dry mustard

⅓ cup (80 ml) extra virgin olive oil

3 tablespoons fresh lemon juice, plus more if needed

1 tablespoon blackstrap molasses

SALAD

14 ounces (6 cups/400 g) Russian Red kale or any other variety of kale, stemmed

1 tablespoon white balsamic vinegar

⅓ cup (75 g) pomegranate arils

1½ tablespoons diced preserved lemon rind

Maldon sea salt flakes

Freshly ground black pepper

Super Seed Blend (page 108), optional

1. To make the dressing: Combine all the ingredients, plus 2 tablespoons water, in a high-speed blender. Blend on high speed, scraping down using a rubber spatula or the blender plunger, until smooth. Adjust the seasoning with more lemon juice, if needed.

2. To make the salad: Tear or chop the kale into roughly 2-inch (5 cm) pieces. Place in a large salad bowl along with the vinegar and massage with clean hands for 1 minute, or until you feel the kale soften.

3. Add the dressing and continue to massage for another minute, to fully coat the kale.

4. Toss with the pomegranate arils and diced preserved lemon. Season with a sprinkle of salt flakes and pepper.

5. Place the kale in a serving bowl and top with Super Seed Blend, if using.

NOTES

This dressing can be made ahead of time and stored in the fridge.

This salad is great on top of a Topped Toast, such as the Pirbright Pea and Mint Toast (page 42).

Beef up this salad with the addition of warm Roasted Vinegar Mushrooms (page 74) and Sumac and Oregano Gigante Beans (page 93), creating a more than satisfying meal and dance of flavors.

TABLE SALAD

There are a million and one things I love about Italy, and many of them are just illustrations of how when you live more slowly and openly, life just gets better. Like with these big salads that arrive to your table, undressed. A glug of beautifully sweet aged balsamic vinegar, additional bright acid, a dash of spicy olive oil—maybe a pinch of herbs, some salt and pepper if you must—are all that you need.

Sure, there is a plethora of phytonutrients in this colorful salad, but for this moment I focus on the actions (or lack thereof) of doing a little less, with a bit more intention and peace.

Makes 4 servings

2 carrots, peeled

5½ ounces (160 g) Belgian endive spears, sliced into rings (3 cups)

5½ ounces (160 g) radicchio leaves, torn (3 cups)

5 tablespoons (40 g) Marcona almonds, roughly chopped

1 tablespoon fresh lemon juice

Maldon sea salt flakes

Freshly ground black pepper

3 tablespoons aged balsamic vinegar

3 tablespoons extra virgin olive oil (use one that you love!)

Fresh oregano, optional

1. Grate the carrots with a box grater or peel into ribbons, using a vegetable peeler, directly into a large salad bowl.

2. Toss the carrots with endive, radicchio, almonds, and lemon juice.

3. Sprinkle a small amount of salt and pepper over the salad and drizzle very lightly with the vinegar and olive oil.

4. In a small side dish, use a spoon to combine the remaining vinegar and olive oil along with oregano, if using, and additional salt and pepper to taste.

NOTES

Fight inflammation with healthy fats and fibrous vegetables. The addition of avocado chunks will up the healthy fats by bringing omega-6 fatty acids to the olive oil's omega-3s.

This salad makes a light and cleansing meal served alongside the Tomato Blitz soup (page 100) for less hungry days or when you need to reset your system.

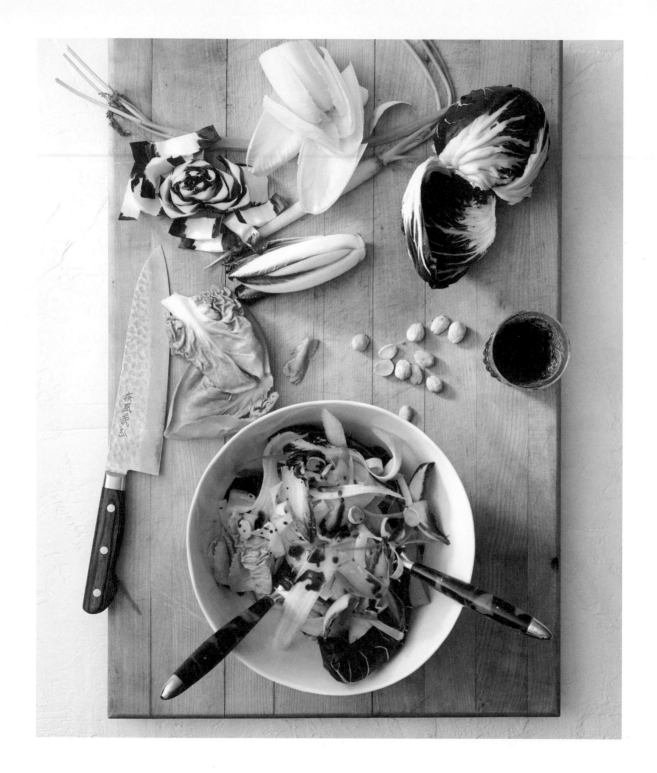

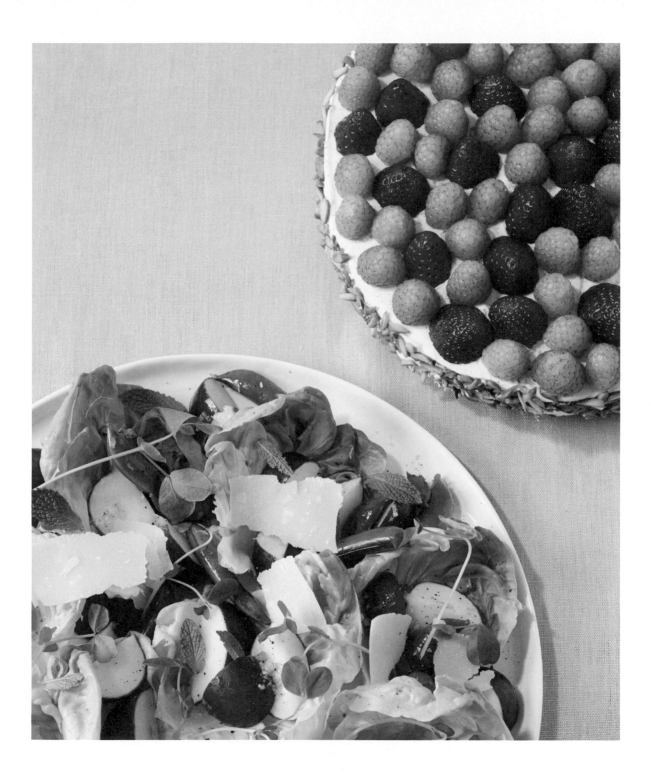

RADISH PEAS PARMESAN

The thoughtful combination of bright, tangy flavors in this salad is classic, the texture so pleasing that it makes me look forward to it every spring when snap peas are fresh and piled everywhere at the market. I will make this out of season, too, as snap peas tend to still be at the store and their sweet bite really does the trick for me. Butter lettuce is so silky and a great complement to all that crunch, though I have been known to go on a lettuce strike and make it without the leafy green addition.

This is another colorful raw vegetable combination full of natural sweetness and phytonutrients. Incorporating spicy vegetables, such as radishes, into your diet helps balance blood sugar levels and aids tremendously in digestion.

This salad is energizing and filling while still being light. Pull this one out of your hat as an easy crowd-pleaser at any meal.

Makes 6 servings

2 ounces (55 g) aged Parmigiano-Reggiano, grated into thin shards (½ cup grated), plus more for sprinkling, optional

1 teaspoon freshly ground black pepper, plus more for sprinkling

½ teaspoon Himalayan pink salt

½ teaspoon grated lemon zest

3 tablespoons fresh lemon juice

2 tablespoons extra virgin olive oil

2 cups (230 g) quartered radishes

2 cups (300 g) snap peas

2 tablespoons torn fresh mint leaves

About 4 ounces (4 cups/110 g) whole butter lettuce leaves, separated

Pea shoots, optional

1. Combine the cheese, pepper, salt, and lemon zest in the bottom of a large bowl.

2. Add the lemon juice and with clean hands massage the cheese and lemon juice together to make a paste.

3. Drizzle in the olive oil and incorporate, using the back of a soupspoon or your hands.

4. Add the radishes and snap peas; toss to coat. Add the mint leaves at the very end.

5. Lay the butter lettuce leaves on your salad platter and then pile radishes and peas into the cups of the leaves.

6. Finish with a dusting of pepper, pea shoots, if using, and additional shards of cheese, if desired.

NOTES

As this salad is full of sturdy vegetables, make it ahead, reserving the more delicate butter lettuce in a separate container to keep for lunch the next day or a future dinner salad.

Pairs well alongside simple soups, Pirbright Pea and Mint Toast (page 42), or Soft Scrambled Eggs with Radishes (page 30).

Use leftover fava beans from the Green Fava Baked Eggs (page 34) as a great base to a meal bowl of beans and snap peas.

HONEYCRISP WHOLE GRAIN AND PECORINO

If every salad has a season, this one's is fall, of course. Will you be judged for making this any time of year? Absolutely not.

Honeycrisp apples came into vogue when I was living in Burlington, Vermont—a place that to this day has some of the best food and baked goods around. One of my oldest friends, Callie, and I would cruise around as an official eating team, grabbing pie and fresh Honeycrisps from the local market and a burrito from New World Tortilla for the road. Clearly those were different eating times, but my love of Honeycrisp apples has remained. A sharp dressing perfectly complements the spicy arugula, while it balances the juicy sweet apples and little nuggets of sheep's milk pecorino cheese.

Salad and greens, simply referencing the inclusion of raw vegetables, does not have to be flavorless or boring, and eating Clean Enough is here to prove that. While this salad is still delicious dairy-free, with a Clean Enough mentality, the smattering of pecorino adds pops of flavor for further satiety. Apples, being high in fiber, keep your mouth entertained as you chew and your digestion in check, all the while tasting juicy and sweet like a treat.

Makes 8 to 10 servings

3 tablespoons cider vinegar

3 tablespoons extra virgin olive oil

3 tablespoons whole grain mustard

2¼ teaspoons freshly ground black pepper

1½ teaspoons raw honey

½ teaspoon Himalayan pink salt

3 tablespoons chopped fresh tarragon leaves

3 Honeycrisp apples (about 1 pound/450 g)

4 ounces (120 g) sheep's milk pecorino, broken into small chunks

12 cups (240 g) baby arugula

1. Whisk together the cider vinegar, olive oil, mustard, pepper, honey, and salt in a salad bowl. Whisk in the tarragon leaves.

2. Cut your Honeycrisp apples into quarters and remove the core by cutting it out at an angle. Slice each quarter into thirds and then chop the apple into haphazard chunks. Place the apple chunks and pecorino in the dressing; toss to coat.

3. Add the arugula on top and toss gently to combine. Serve immediately.

――――――

NOTES

Pair this with chopped soft-boiled egg (see page 27) and Sweet-and-Sour Green Beans (page 76) for my take on a New England Cobb salad.

Fall flavors combine with the addition of a bowl of Fermented Garlic and Squash Soup (page 99) or Velvet Beet soup (page 101).

HAZELNUT ARUGULA

Toasted hazelnuts pack an excellent flavor punch in a wide array of dishes, sweet and savory alike. In my love of supersimple, and simply dressed, greens, the addition of warm toasted hazelnut to this vinaigrette elevates the whole thing, rounding out a meal to savor. These greens are a great topper to a layered bowl of beans and Romesco (page 113), adding a spicy green kick. Arugula has a distinct peppery flavor that is not as sharp as, say, mizuna, lending itself well to a variety of salads, with its fairly sturdy yet delicate nature.

Makes 6 servings

⅔ cup (90 g) whole hazelnuts, skin on

¼ cup (60 ml) extra virgin olive oil

Juice of 1 lemon

1 teaspoon Himalayan pink salt

½ teaspoon freshly ground black pepper

7 ounces (10 cups/200 g) baby arugula

1. Preheat the oven to 300°F (150°C) convection. Place the hazelnuts on an unlined baking sheet and roast in the oven for 15 minutes, allowing the nuts to toast slowly and evenly.

2. Let the loose skins of the nuts fall off and discard. While they're still hot, crush the hazelnuts on the pan with the back of a small sauté pan. (Some of the hazelnuts will powder while other pieces will remain whole.)

3. Place the hot crushed hazelnuts in a large salad bowl along with the olive oil, lemon juice, and salt. Macerate the nuts with a spoon by stirring for a minute, flavoring the oil and lemon. Add the black pepper.

4. Pile the arugula on top of the dressing and toss just before serving.

NOTES

Salad on top of soup can be and is delicious, and this salad is a perfect complement to wilt on top of a bowl of Healing Congee (page 104), Fermented Garlic and Squash Soup (page 99), Velvet Beet soup (page 101), and even cold Tomato Blitz (page 100).

The salad also complements Pesto (page 118) and served alongside the Mid-August Lunch (page 56) further livens up the dish.

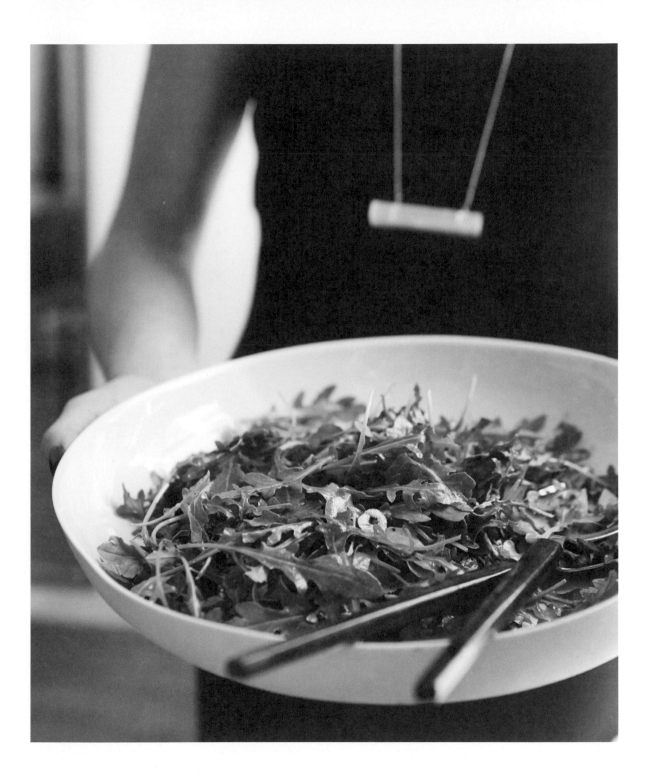

MID-AUGUST LUNCH

I haphazardly made this original salad, kind of like the way a hot and lazy August afternoon sneaks up on you and ends either in an impromptu nap or some memorable evening, always unplanned. It showcases all my favorite loves: Pesto (which I pour on almost everything except pasta, on which I prefer tomatoes), hearty gigante beans, and seared zucchini. This salad is full of fibrous zucchini, which, while not nutrient-dense, adds a great volume, texture, and flavor. Pesto, a great tool for your Clean pantry, does not need to involve dairy, instead relying heavily on medicinal, cleansing, high-flavor herbs, heart-healthy nuts, and bright vitamin C–packed lemon. Goes down easy like a glass of Chianti.

Makes 8 servings

4 zucchini (a little over 1 pound/ 500 g)

3 tablespoons extra virgin olive oil

1 tablespoon + 1 teaspoon fresh lemon juice

Pinch Himalayan pink salt

Pinch freshly ground black pepper

2 cups (280 g) cooked and rinsed gigante beans

½ cup (110 g) Pesto (page 118)

¼ cup (30 g) raw pine nuts

1. Using a vegetable peeler or mandoline, cut two of the raw zucchini lengthwise into thin ribbons. Toss with 1 tablespoon of the olive oil plus the lemon juice, salt, and pepper; set aside.

2. Cut the remaining two zucchini in half lengthwise and then cut into haphazard ¾-inch (2 cm) half-moon chunks, the more haphazard the better. Heat the remaining 2 tablespoons olive oil in a heavy-bottomed skillet over medium-high heat. Add the zucchini chunks and sauté to caramelize for 4 minutes. Add the gigante beans and continue to sauté for 2 minutes. Remove the pan from the heat and fold in the Pesto.

3. Toss the raw and warm zucchini mixtures together, transfer to a serving bowl, and top with the pine nuts.

VARIATION

Instead of adding warm Pesto to the caramelized zucchini, try combining the Pesto with the cooked gigantes in a food processor and pulsing until smooth. Spread the beans at the bottom of a bowl or platter and top with the raw and caramelized zucchini tossed together. Finish with the pine nuts.

NOTE

You can purchase precooked gigante beans, or quick-soak and cook them from dried (see Sumac and Oregano Gigante Beans, page 93).

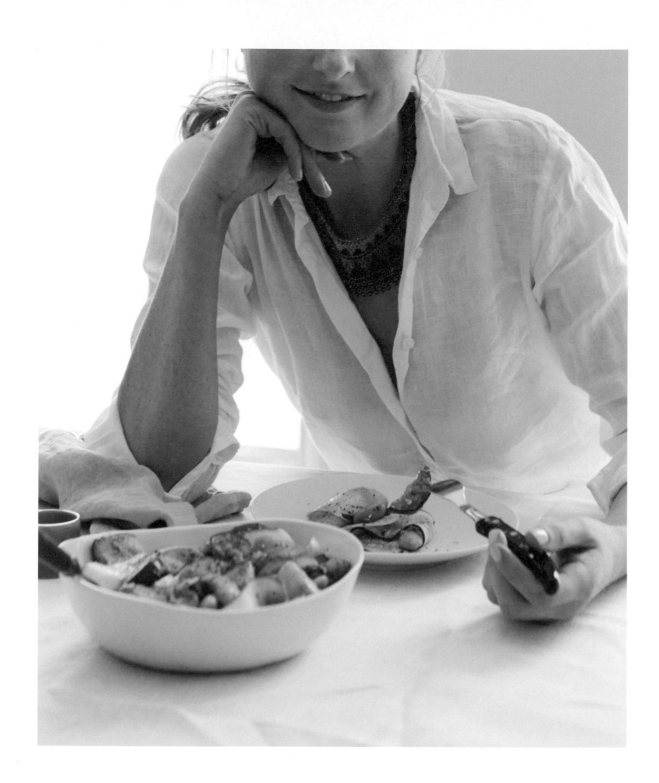

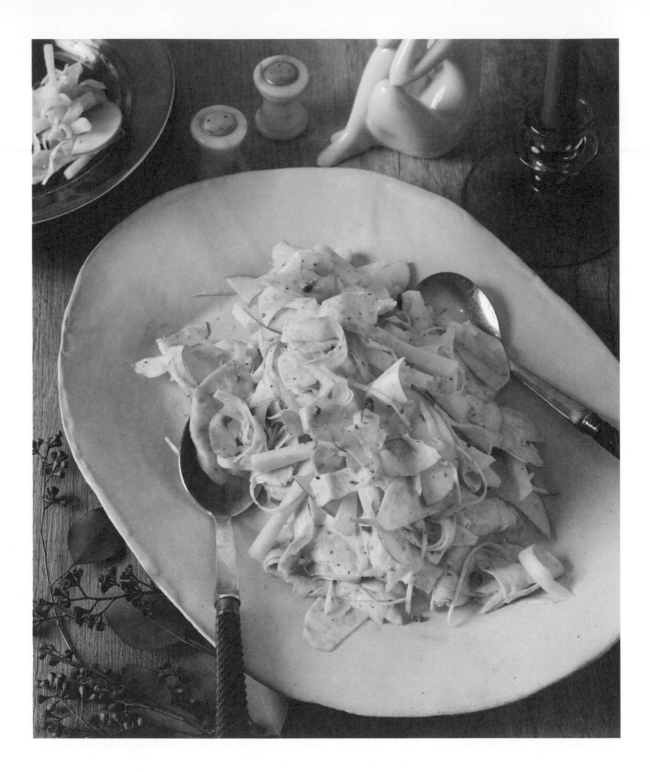

CELERY ROOT AND JICAMA

My best friend, Sam, and I have known each other for what feels like a lifetime. She is like a sister to me, and I can always count on her (to eat this salad!). Love is not enough to describe her feelings about this salad. The time it was first served to her was at one of the best dinner parties I have hosted thus far with my friend and charity cochair Walton. The theme was the South of France and we delivered, complete with the famous pommes Aligot (read: potato fondue), macaroons, croquembouche, and this salad. Clean, classic, and full of prebiotic fiber, essential for feeding healthy probiotic bacteria in your gut, as well as calcium and potassium, this salad gets better as it becomes *tired*, meaning I like it just as much the next day as I do freshly tossed.

Makes 6 servings

1 garlic clove, peeled

1 large pasture-raised egg yolk

1½ teaspoons Himalayan pink salt

1½ teaspoons freshly ground black pepper

¼ teaspoon grated lemon zest

2 tablespoons extra virgin olive oil

1 tablespoon + 1 teaspoon fresh lemon juice

1 tablespoon Dijon mustard

2 teaspoons capers, drained, rinsed, and chopped

1 celery root (about 11 ounces/300 g)

1 organic Granny Smith apple

1 jicama (about 9 ounces/250 g)

1. Grate the garlic directly into a salad bowl. Whisk in the egg yolk, salt, pepper, and lemon zest.

2. Whisking continuously, slowly stream in the olive oil. The mixture should become thick and emulsified.

3. Whisk in the lemon juice, mustard, and chopped capers.

4. Peel the celery root and cut in half. Begin cutting the celery root halves on a mandoline, creating thin half-moon slices. It is important for the celery root to be sliced as paper thin as you are able to achieve.

5. Cut the apple into quarters and core, using a knife at an angle. Then slice the quarters into thin slices, less than ⅛ inch (3 mm) thick.

6. Peel the jicama and cut into batons ¼ inch (6 mm) thick.

7. Toss the celery root, apple, and jicama together and add to the dressing. Toss to combine well.

8. Serve immediately at room temperature—or to enjoy as a tired salad, chill to serve at a later date. The salad keeps for a day and a half.

NOTES

Celery root is a rough and often dirty root vegetable. Wash it well and trim away the sides before slicing for salad. Some celery roots need to be trimmed more, resulting in a smaller usable vegetable than anticipated. If necessary, purchase an additional one so that you have enough usable product for the salad.

This salad is excellent with Longevity Mushroom Toast (page 39).

MANGO SAUERKRAUT SLAW

Think about an amazing taco with fresh cabbage on top. Sounds like a perfect postbeach afternoon snack, right? Add some mango and we're in heaven.

Back to reality, swap out some of the cabbage for sauerkraut and you get the gut-loving umami heaven that is this slaw. Sauerkraut (fermented cabbage) is unbelievably easy to make (see page 112 for proof). In a pinch, you can buy sauerkraut (I much prefer the red cabbage variety) to add to this salad. Either way, the result is a delicious taco topping, a superflavorful side salad or side dish, or a great bowl topper. You can do a lot with this slaw—but do not be surprised if eating it right out of the bowl is enough.

Makes 4 servings

½ teaspoon grated lime zest

2 tablespoons fresh lime juice

1 teaspoon coconut oil

½ teaspoon Rooster Sauce (page 116)

¼ teaspoon ground cumin

¼ teaspoon Himalayan pink salt

¼ teaspoon freshly ground black pepper

5 ounces (140 g) fresh green cabbage, fresh and shredded into ¼-inch (6 mm) pieces (1 cup)

½ (5-ounce/140 g) mango, peeled, seeded, and cut into ¼-inch (6 mm) pieces

1 cup (40 g) fresh cilantro leaves

1½ ounces (40 g) red onion, sliced paper thin (¼ cup), optional

1 cup (140 g) Kraut (page 112)

1. To make the dressing, combine the lime zest and juice, coconut oil, Rooster Sauce, cumin, salt, and pepper in a small bowl.

2. Toss together the shredded green cabbage, mango, cilantro, and onion, if using, in a large bowl.

3. Pour the dressing over the cabbage mixture and toss gently to coat.

4. Add the Kraut and toss gently again, as the sauerkraut will stain both the cabbage and mango purple.

5. Serve immediately, or store in the fridge for up to a day.

NOTES

Toast and fill an organic corn, cassava, or almond flour tortilla with Guacamole (page 111) and Midnight Carrots (page 78), topping with a generous portion of this slaw, for a great plant-based lunch, snack, or casual dinner.

If you have not prepared the Rooster Sauce, you can use an organic sriracha sauce; be sure to check that there are no added preservatives or refined sugars.

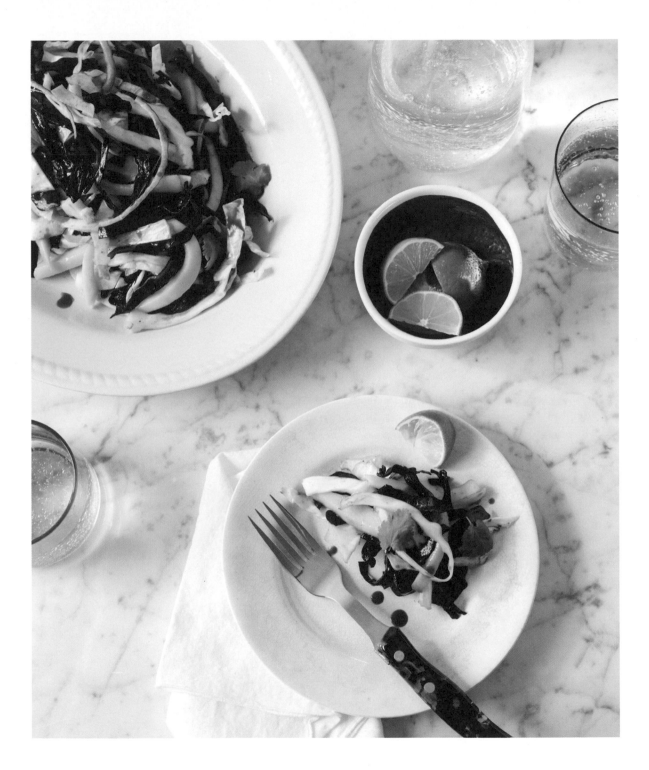

EAT THE RAINBOW SALAD

Oh, the dance of flavors in this salad. I am a big fan of the earthy grated sweet potato mingling with the sweet and juicy grated or peeled carrots. A whisper of tahini adds a bit of creaminess to the otherwise vinegary concoction, rounded out with chamomile-scented pickled raisins and bright fresh herbs. Despite its being a raw salad, this is something that feels almost soft and unctuous, deeply satisfying while cleansing and vitamin-packed.

Makes 8 servings

PICKLED TEA RAISINS (SEE NOTES)

¾ cup (180 ml) white balsamic vinegar

2 tablespoons dried chamomile tea flowers

1 cup (180 g) organic golden raisins

1 cup (180 g) organic dark raisins

SALAD

About 11 ounces (300 g) raw sweet potato, peeled and grated on a box grater (2 cups)

2 tablespoons extra virgin olive oil

2 tablespoons tahini paste

2 tablespoons white wine vinegar

1 teaspoon ground coriander seeds

1 teaspoon ground cumin

½ teaspoon Himalayan pink salt

About 11 ounces (300 g) carrots, grated or peeled into long ribbons (2 cups)

2 tablespoons thinly sliced scallion (green part only)

1 cup (60 g) fresh parsley leaves, roughly chopped

½ cup (20 g) fresh cilantro leaves, roughly chopped

Super Seed Blend (page 108), optional

1. To make the Pickled Tea Raisins: Place the vinegar, chamomile, and ¾ cup (180 ml) water in a small saucepan and bring to a simmer. Turn off the heat and allow to steep for 5 minutes.

2. Combine the raisins in a heatproof bowl. Strain the liquid and pour over the raisins. Place in a container in the fridge to cool and hydrate. Store in the cooking vinegar for up to 2 weeks, squeezing the raisins of excess liquid before use.

3. To make the salad: Place the grated sweet potato in ice water to release excess starch. Squeeze and pat dry on a clean kitchen towel.

4. Whisk together the olive oil, tahini, vinegar, coriander seeds, cumin, and salt in the bottom of a salad bowl.

5. Add the carrots, scallion, sweet potato, and 1 cup (160 g) of the Pickled Tea Raisins. Toss to combine well. Add the parsley and cilantro leaves and toss again.

6. Serve immediately or store in the fridge to hold. Before serving, top with Super Seed Blend, if using.

NOTES

You will have leftover Pickled Tea Raisins (this recipe makes 3 cups/300 g), which I love on a good bread with a schmear of ricotta, some honey, and walnuts.

This is an excellent side dish paired with the Gentle Lentils (page 90) for a very grounding meal that could be useful during transitional times.

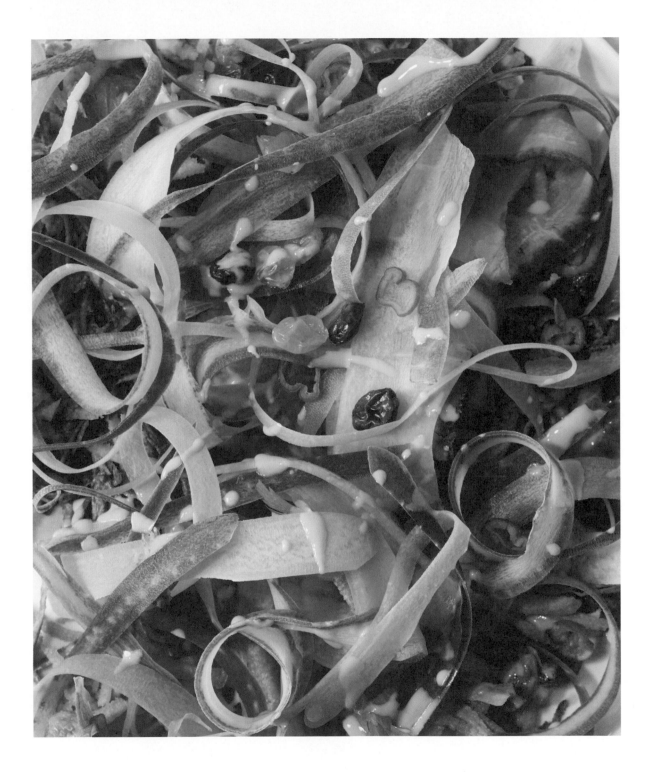

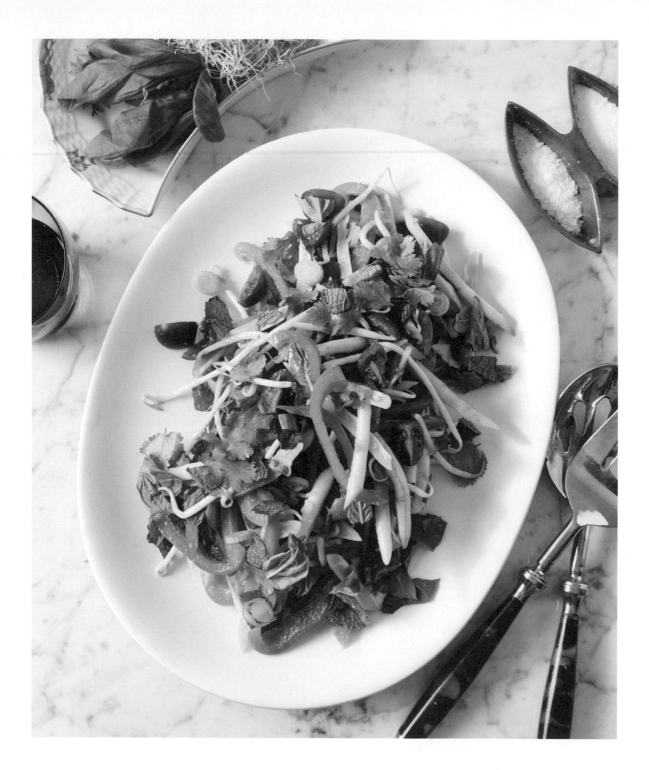

BRIGHT BEAN SPROUT SALAD

I have been teaching after-school cooking with Goals4Kids at P.S. 171 in Harlem for a decade, where once a week we prepare a meal together and then sit down to eat and chat. I feebly try to be brought up to speed on what is cool in the world of adolescents, but I impress them (I think) with how easy it can be to make healthy foods, and how enjoyable the eating-together part can be.

This salad, in one iteration or another, has made an appearance at school more than once over the years. The real secret is the addition of rice "flour" (read: ground rice), which creates something absolutely creamy and slightly textured in the dressing. But the most important thing about the origins of this salad? It's a precursor to the never-missed Goal4Kids dessert.

Makes 8 servings

2 large yellow bell peppers

7 ounces (2 cups/200 g) yellow wax beans

2 tablespoons + 2 teaspoons (40 ml) rice wine vinegar

1 tablespoon ground rice flour

2 teaspoons Bragg Liquid Aminos

2 teaspoons Rooster Sauce (page 116)

2 teaspoons toasted sesame oil

1 teaspoon grated fresh ginger

½ teaspoon grated garlic

½ teaspoon Dijon mustard

About 11 ounces (300 g) bean sprouts (3 cups)

12 Kumato or cherry tomatoes, halved

½ cup (20 g) basil leaves, cut into ribbons

½ cup (50 g) mint leaves, roughly chopped

½ cup (20 g) whole cilantro leaves

½ cup (30 g) whole parsley leaves

4 scallions (green parts only), sliced into thin disks (heaping ¼ cup/25 g)

Lime wedges

1. Cut the bell peppers in half, seed, then slice lengthwise into very thin slices.

2. Trim the ends of the beans and then carefully cut them in half lengthwise, then in half again widthwise.

3. Whisk together the vinegar, rice flour, liquid aminos, Rooster Sauce, sesame oil, ginger, garlic, and mustard in a salad bowl.

4. Add the bean sprouts, bell pepper, beans, and tomatoes. Toss to combine. Add the herbs and scallions and toss well.

5. Serve the salad with fresh lime wedges.

NOTES

Bean sprouts are an excellent source of protein, making this a complete yet carb-conscious meal. For added energy, enjoy with a portion of Miso Brown Rice (page 82) or Eastern Medicine Health Rice (page 87) along with a handful of almonds or organic shelled soybeans.

This salad definitely keeps your system moving, as it is all raw fibrous vegetables with a generous amount of liver-cleansing parsley and cilantro.

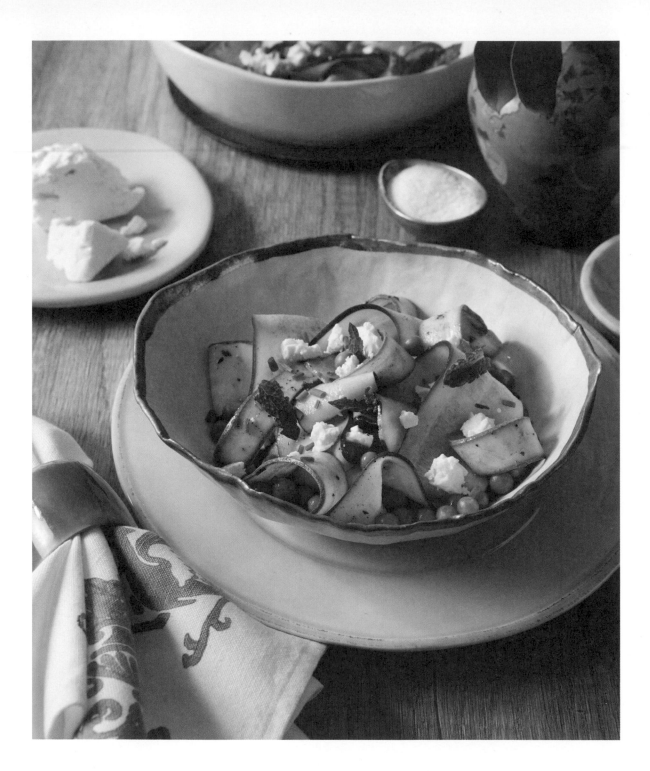

ZUCCHINI AND SPRING PEA MACHINE

I am not so much a noodle girl as I am a ribbon lady. Ribbons of anything are poetic, whereas noodles have a definite connotation that I like to save for pasta arrabiatta on a Sunday. The poetry of these zucchini ribbons comes from the harmony of their creamy texture with pickled dressing, sweet peas, and salty feta.

Makes 4 servings

⅔ cup (160 ml) white wine vinegar

2 tablespoons raw honey

2 teaspoons ground turmeric

1 teaspoon celery seeds

1 teaspoon whole yellow mustard seeds

½ teaspoon dried mint

½ teaspoon ground cumin

2 zucchini (9 ounces/250 g)

1⅓ cups (200 g) fresh peas (see Notes)

2 tablespoons extra virgin olive oil

2 tablespoons finely minced fresh chives

2 tablespoons roughly chopped fresh mint leaves

½ teaspoon Himalayan pink salt

½ teaspoon freshly ground black pepper

1 ounce (30 g) goat's milk feta (3 tablespoons crumbled)

1. Combine the vinegar, honey, turmeric, celery seeds, mustard, dried mint, and cumin in a small saucepan. Bring to a simmer and then turn off the heat.

2. Using a mandoline, slice the zucchini lengthwise into thin, long ribbons. Lay the zucchini flat in a shallow baking dish and pour the vinegar mixture directly on top.

3. Place in the fridge for 20 minutes to cool and tenderize, flipping the zucchini over once, halfway through.

4. Meanwhile, bring about 3 cups (720 ml) water to a boil in a small saucepan. Add the peas and blanch for 30 seconds. Drain immediately to stop the cooking process and then allow to cool.

5. Drain the zucchini well, gently patting off the excess moisture with a paper towel. You can save the pickling liquid separately to prepare an additional salad at a later date.

6. Toss the zucchini with the olive oil, chives, mint, salt, and pepper.

7. Gently toss in the peas and top with the crumbled feta.

NOTE

Frozen peas work well; simply allow them to thaw before adding them to the dressed zucchini, skipping over the step of blanching them.

SESAME CUCUMBER SALAD

Don't let the simple name of this recipe belie its layered complexity. I have almost completely stopped cooking with standard and even the less seedy English cucumbers as a result of discovering the petite Persian cucumber, which is loaded with hydration and crunch. I tend to have Persian cucumbers around as a positive snack, as a smart option for such dips as guacamole, to toss in a salad, and to keep on hand for this recipe. This salad stands on its own and is also excellent to top hearty bowls of nourishing bean and millet–enriched Eastern Medicine Health Rice (page 87) or Healing Congee (page 104). The addition of this cucumber salad leaves me satisfied and clean.

Makes 4 servings

2 tablespoons brown rice vinegar

2 teaspoons grated fresh ginger

1 tablespoon plain sesame oil

½ teaspoon toasted sesame oil

½ teaspoon Bragg Liquid Aminos

9 ounces (250 g) Persian cucumbers (about 4), sliced into ¼-inch (6 mm) disks

2 teaspoons black sesame seeds

1. Whisk together the vinegar, ginger, sesame oils, and liquid aminos in a medium bowl.

2. Add the cucumber slices to the bowl and toss together. Sprinkle with the black sesame seeds.

3. Serve immediately or store in the fridge to retain crispiness until ready to serve.

PREPARED VEGETABLES

I believe there is a fair amount of confusion around raw versus cooked vegetables and what is deemed to be healthier. To begin, vegetables, as a whole, contribute to your health without question, whether raw or cooked. They are real-food, single ingredients, full of vitamins and minerals absolutely essential for your bodily functions. To complete the circle, you need to add to your individual mix of healthy fats and clean protein, with the vegetables either acting as or complementing a source of carbohydrates.

Now for the matter of raw versus cooked and whether raw is healthier than prepared. Some vegetables taste better raw and others, cooked. Many vegetables are easier on your digestion when lightly steamed, sautéed, or blanched, as the fiber is easier to break down. Consider raw greens and salads to be light and energetic, hydrating, full of live enzymes, acting as a broom to your digestive system. Prepared or cooked vegetables, while still full of fiber, vitamins, and minerals, are more grounding to your body and digestive system. I like to think of eating vegetables throughout the day in a progression. If given the choice for (my) best digestion, I like to taper eating raw vegetables as the day progresses, ending with (mostly) cooked because, as mentioned, they tend to be easier on digestion, which is helpful as you slow down at day's end.

These prepared vegetables are (almost) all great for cooking multiple portions of to have on hand throughout the week. They can stand on their own or become a component to a meal, a bowl, or part of a spread when cooking for others. The latter is the foundation for my entertaining prowess. Paired with various condiments from the pantry section, there is enough in this section to go around.

BRAISED BLUE ZONE GREENS

Want to live to forever? Eat braised bitter greens. I am not a doctor, but I do pay attention to what different cultures eat around the world—specifically in blue zones, where people live the longest, with the highest quality of life, and eat lots of greens. Spinach, collard greens, choy sum, all the kale, and mustard greens can be used in this recipe interchangeably. The family of greens contains a host of vitamins and minerals, along with cleansing properties that are excellent for your kidney and liver. Make each forkful a toast to a long, happy life spent eating greens.

Makes 6 servings

9 ounces (255 g) Swiss chard

2 garlic cloves, peeled and smashed

1 shallot, sliced thinly

1 tablespoon grated fresh ginger

1 tablespoon plain sesame oil

9 ounces (255 g) chicory, roughly chopped (3 cups)

3 ounces (85 g) escarole, roughly chopped (2 cups)

3 ounces (85 g) lacinto or another green kale, stemmed and chopped into 2-inch (5 cm) ribbons (2 cups)

About 1½ ounces (45 g) dandelion greens, roughly chopped into 2-inch (5 cm) pieces (1 cup)

2 cups (475 ml) unsalted organic vegetable stock

1 tablespoon Bragg Liquid Aminos

1 tablespoon rice wine vinegar

1½ teaspoons toasted sesame oil

1 teaspoon Himalayan pink salt

½ teaspoon freshly ground black pepper

3 tablespoons fresh oregano leaves

1½ teaspoons white sesame seeds

Lemon wedges

Super Seed Blend (page 108), optional

1. Remove the stems from the chard and roughly chop the leaves into 2-inch (5 cm) pieces (3 cups). Reserve 2½ ounces (75 g) of the stems, sliced into ½-inch (5 cm) pieces (1 cup).

2. Combine the garlic, shallot, ginger, chard stems, and plain sesame oil in a large flat-bottomed skillet with a lid. Sauté over medium heat until translucent, 6 minutes.

3. Increase the heat to high and pile in the greens, including the chard leaves. They will take up a lot of volume but will wilt down. Sauté for 5 minutes.

4. Add the vegetable stock, liquid aminos, and vinegar to the wilted greens, lowering the heat to low and placing a lid on the skillet to simmer for 10 minutes, further softening the greens; the coloring will darken slightly. Then remove the lid and continue to simmer, reducing the liquid for 15 minutes.

5. When half of the liquid has evaporated and the greens have fully softened, remove the pan from the heat and add the toasted sesame oil, salt, and pepper.

6. Place in a serving dish or serve directly from the pan with oregano and sesame seeds sprinkled on top and lemon wedges on the side. Top with Super Seed Blend, if desired.

7. Alternatively, if not serving immediately, omit the seed toppings and store in the fridge as a prepped vegetable for your week, reheating in a sauté pan as needed and then topping with the oregano and seeds.

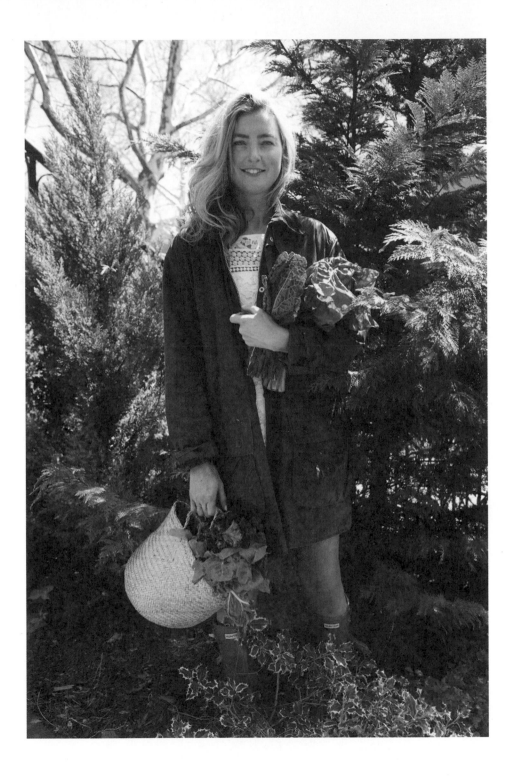

CHARRED PUMPKIN SEED BROCCOLINI

I love simply steamed broccoli, the purest version of Clean Enough, and when I am in the mood for more flavor, this pumpkin seed–coated roasted broccolini is exquisite and nutrient-dense. Pumpkin seeds are powerful, containing inflammation-reducing omega-3 fatty acids, progesterone-boosting zinc for hormone regulation, and a significant amount of protein. Broccolini is a powerhouse full of calcium, iron, and protein as well. Labne acts as the glue in this recipe and adds an additional layer of calcium. I treat the broccolini at times like my version of kale chips, albeit much easier to digest as it is not completely dried. Baby broccoli is more tender than regular broccoli crowns, requiring less trimming of the stalks before cooking.

Makes 6 servings

¼ cup (60 g) Labne (page 109)

2 tablespoons extra virgin olive oil

½ teaspoon Himalayan pink salt

½ teaspoon freshly ground black pepper

13 ounces (375 g/2 bunches) baby broccolini, ends slightly trimmed

½ cup (60 g) raw pumpkin seeds, ground

1 lemon, cut in half

½ teaspoon grated lemon zest

1. Preheat the oven to 450°F (230°C) convection.

2. Combine the Labne, olive oil, salt, and pepper in a large bowl.

3. Add the broccolini and massage to coat well. Add the pumpkin seeds and toss to coat well.

4. Place on an unlined half sheet pan, spreading out to allow each piece of broccolini to cook evenly. Place the lemon halves on one side of the sheet pan so that they can roast while the broccolini chars.

5. Roast in the oven for 15 to 20 minutes, until crispy and deep golden.

6. Remove from the oven and sprinkle the broccolini with lemon zest.

7. Serve immediately with a squeeze of roasted lemon or store in the fridge as a prepped vegetable for your week, reheating in the oven to re-crisp.

VARIATIONS

To stay inspired, try making this dish using a variety of vegetables that you enjoy roasted. Maintain the same baking temperature and watch for doneness, or a slight golden of the pumpkin seeds and tenderness of the vegetable. Cauliflower, parsnips, carrots, sweet potatoes, green beans, and kabocha squash all can evolve with a coating of tangy Labne, and heart-healthy, crunchy pumpkin seeds.

NOTES

This vegetable is a great topper to the Eastern Medicine Health Rice (page 87), Miso Brown Rice (page 82), and Coconut Oil Crispy Rice (page 97).

The broccolini is also a great vehicle for a dip, such as the Tzatziki (page 109), Romesco (page 113), or Pesto (page 118).

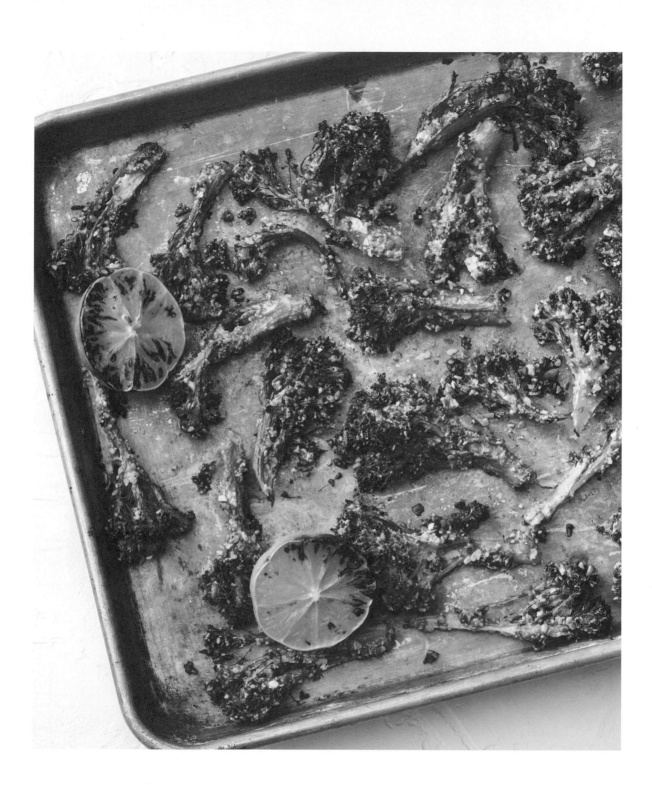

ROASTED VINEGAR MUSHROOMS

Not what you would expect from a roasted mushroom, this vegetable dish is more of the tapas persuasion, delicious on its own and also a tremendous supplement to a variety of the Clean recipes, adding a heartiness, a bright acidic flavor, and an array of minerals.

Makes 6 servings

⅓ cup (80 ml) aged balsamic vinegar

2 tablespoons sherry vinegar

1 tablespoon extra virgin olive oil

1 garlic clove, peeled and minced

½ teaspoon crushed red pepper flakes

½ teaspoon Himalayan pink salt

½ teaspoon freshly ground black pepper

2½ cups (190 g) baby portobello mushrooms

2½ cups (190 g) white button mushrooms, cleaned

1 cup (75 g) shiitake mushrooms, cleaned

10 thyme sprigs

½ cup (30 g) fresh parsley, roughly chopped

1. Preheat the oven to 400°F (200°C) convection.

2. Combine the balsamic and sherry vinegar, olive oil, garlic, red pepper flakes, salt, and black pepper in a large bowl.

3. Add the whole mushrooms and thyme sprigs. Toss well to combine and allow to sit for 10 minutes to macerate.

4. Place the mushrooms on an unlined half sheet pan or in a cast-iron skillet and roast in the oven for 30 to 40 minutes, until tender and browned with the vinegar reduced.

5. Remove from the oven and toss with the parsley.

6. Serve immediately or store in the fridge as a prepped vegetable for your week.

NOTES

Serve alongside Little Black Dressed Greens (page 47) and Peruvian Quinoa (page 86) for a balanced meal.

Top the Kale and Preserved Lemon Caesar (page 48) with the mushrooms and serve with a side of Pesto (page 118) and toast.

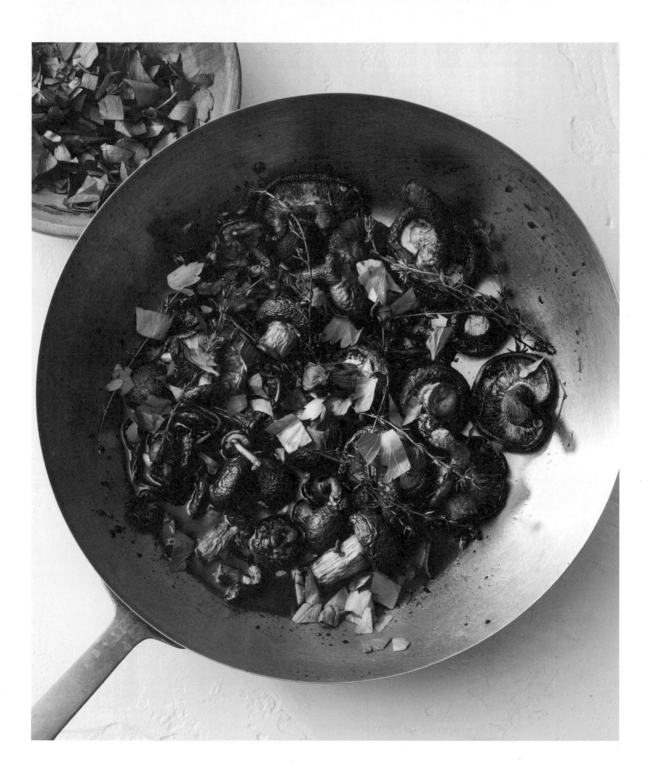

SWEET-AND-SOUR GREEN BEANS

All vegetables must be cooked "properly," my Uncle Robbie would say, sage advice that comes to mind most every time I cook, but especially when I make green beans. This simple vegetable was a staple side dish present at almost every meal we all shared while visiting Halifax as a kid, where he taught me a Clean Enough constant: the care of simple ingredients. His biggest secret: Blanch these green beans before searing them in the cast-iron skillet. The resulting texture is perfectly tender, caramelized, and delicious. Tamarind is a sweet-and-sour root commonly used in cuisines around the world, especially those known for their regional curries. Pungent sage—a medicinal herb whose literal meaning is "saved"—has been linked to mental clarity. Paired with earthy hazelnuts, this dish is what I'd call proper eating—and nothing short of magic.

Makes 6 servings

1 pound (6 cups/450 g) green beans

2 tablespoons fresh sage leaves

2 tablespoons raw hazelnuts

½ teaspoon Himalayan pink salt

½ teaspoon freshly ground black pepper

2 teaspoons plain sesame oil

2 teaspoons organic tamarind concentrate

1. Bring a medium pot of water to a boil. Meanwhile, trim the green bean ends. Place beans in the boiling water to blanch for 1 minute, or until they just turn bright green. Immediately drain the beans and rinse under cool water.

2. To prepare the topping, chop the sage leaves and hazelnuts together on a cutting board. Place the nut mixture in a dry cast-iron skillet over medium heat and toast, stirring, for 3 to 4 minutes, until golden. Immediately transfer the nut mixture to a bowl, season with salt and pepper, and set aside.

3. Heat the sesame oil in the same cast-iron skillet over high heat. Add the blanched green beans and sear for 1 minute. Add the tamarind paste and sear for another minute, or until caramelized. Finally, toss the green beans with the nut mixture.

4. Serve immediately or store in the fridge as a prepped vegetable for your week.

VARIATIONS

To stay inspired, try this with other vegetables that are prepared well when sautéed. Bok choy does not need to be blanched and can be cut into quarters lengthwise, pan-seared until tender with the addition of tamarind, and finished with the sage and hazelnuts.

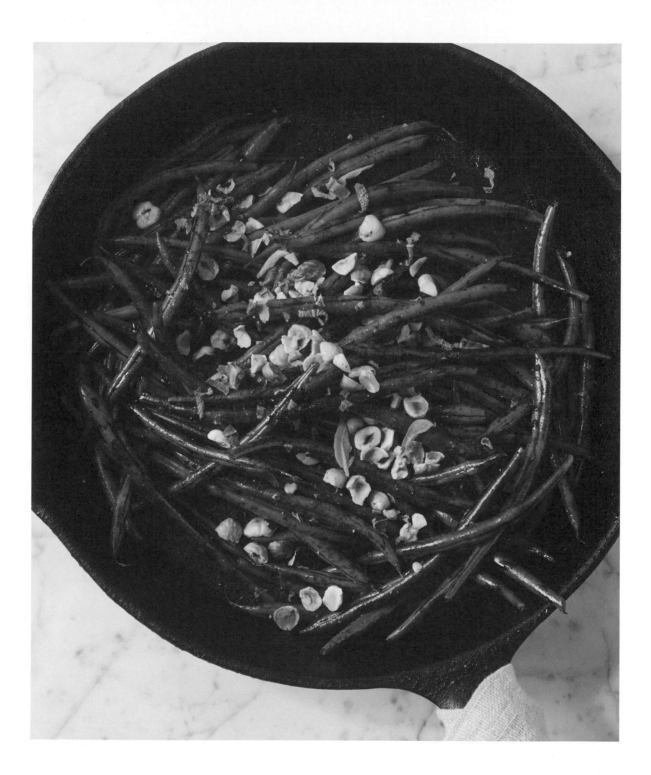

MIDNIGHT CARROTS

The first time I made these carrots, I was hosting some of my girlfriends for our monthly supper club. It was my turn to host the group and cook, but this time I was leaving for Beijing on a two-week solo work trip and was typically overcommitted and exasperated. Yet the evening turned out to be pretty spectacular, complete with a table draped in green velvet running down the center of my cozy studio, spread with about ten versions of veggies with different deceptively simple preparations.

Fermented black garlic is fragrant and sweet without the spicy bite of raw garlic, yet with all the antimicrobial and medicinal benefits. It simply needs to be blitzed together with a bit of oil to make a marinade, resulting in a sweet, garlicky roasted carrot that is nothing short of divine and Clean on a moment's notice.

Makes 6 to 8 servings

2 tablespoons plain sesame oil

4 black garlic cloves

2 tablespoons blackstrap molasses

1 teaspoon Himalayan pink salt

1 teaspoon freshly ground black pepper

2 pounds (905 g) heirloom carrots, peeled

1 orange

1. Preheat the oven to 425°F (220°C) convection.

2. Combine the sesame oil, garlic, molasses, salt, and pepper in a blender or food processor. Blend until smooth, add a tablespoon of water if necessary.

3. Massage the carrots with the marinade and place on a parchment-lined half sheet pan.

4. Roast the carrots in the oven for 35 minutes, turning halfway through.

5. When the carrots are tender and browned, remove from the oven and zest the orange directly on top of the hot carrots.

6. Serve immediately or store in the fridge as a prepped vegetable for your week.

NOTES

If the carrots are thicker than ¾ inch (2 cm) in diameter, slice them in half lengthwise, to allow for faster roasting.

This is an excellent side dish or bowl topper. The flavors pair well with the Sweet-and-Sour Green Beans (page 76) , Miso Brown Rice (page 82), Eastern Medicine Health Rice (page 87), or Blistered Miso Sweet Potatoes (page 83), for a bright finish.

Pair these with the Mango Sauerkraut Slaw (page 60) and Guacamole (page 111) to have as a plant-based taco.

Heirloom carrots are a multicolored variety with the same sweet carrot flavor. Standard organic orange carrots will also work well.

BLACK EGGPLANT

I knew little to nothing about Persian cuisine until a few years ago but was quick to connect to it as it's packed with the most ancient applications of what we now call superfoods. Healing spices without the intensity of Indian cuisine, fresh herbs on and in everything, nuts soaked for easier digestion, you name it; it was earmarked. Plus, every dish I came across was thoughtfully prepared through and through, including this inspired variation on traditional *koresht*, or stew. While this dish does not appear Clean like a bowl of dressed greens, it is the epitome of being just Clean Enough, with healthy fats, healing spices, robust vegetables, and gut-friendly fermented bacteria.

Share this dish, eat it with beautiful Coconut Oil Crispy Rice (page 97), and be who you are.

Makes 6 to 8 servings

8 ounces (about 1¼ cups/225 g) organic crushed Italian tomatoes

½ cup (50 g) raw walnuts, toasted and then ground

1 teaspoon ground Ceylon cinnamon

1½ tablespoons extra virgin olive oil

1 small yellow onion, peeled and cut into thin slices

1 garlic clove, peeled and cut into thin slices

¼ cup (60 g) pomegranate molasses

1 tablespoon white miso paste

1 teaspoon Himalayan pink salt

¾ teaspoon freshly ground black pepper

1¾ pounds (800 g) Japanese eggplants (about 5 eggplants)

½ cup (50 g) fresh mint, chopped

½ cup (110 g) pomegranate arils

½ cup (120 ml) Tzatziki (page 109)

1. Turn the broiler on in the oven to preheat.

2. Combine the crushed tomatoes, 2 cups (480 ml) water, and the walnuts and cinnamon in a medium saucepan. Bring to a simmer over medium heat and cook for 20 minutes, to release the fat from walnuts.

3. Heat 1 tablespoon of the olive oil in a medium sauté pan over medium heat. Add the onion and garlic slices and brown for 15 minutes.

4. Transfer the tomato mixture and browned onion and garlic, along with the pomegranate molasses, miso paste, and ½ teaspoon each of the salt and pepper to a high-powered blender and puree until smooth.

5. Cut the eggplants in half lengthwise and rub the cut side with the remaining 1½ teaspoons olive oil, ½ teaspoon salt, and ¼ teaspoon pepper.

6. Place the eggplants on an unlined half sheet pan and place under the broiler for 10 minutes per side to char. Remove the eggplant from the oven and turn on the convection oven to 375°F (190°C).

7. Pour the tomato mixture into a shallow casserole dish and submerge the eggplant in the sauce, cut side up. Place the eggplant in the oven and bake for 30 minutes, or until bubbly and golden.

8. Remove the eggplant from the oven and top with the mint and pomegranate arils. Serve the Tzatziki on the side.

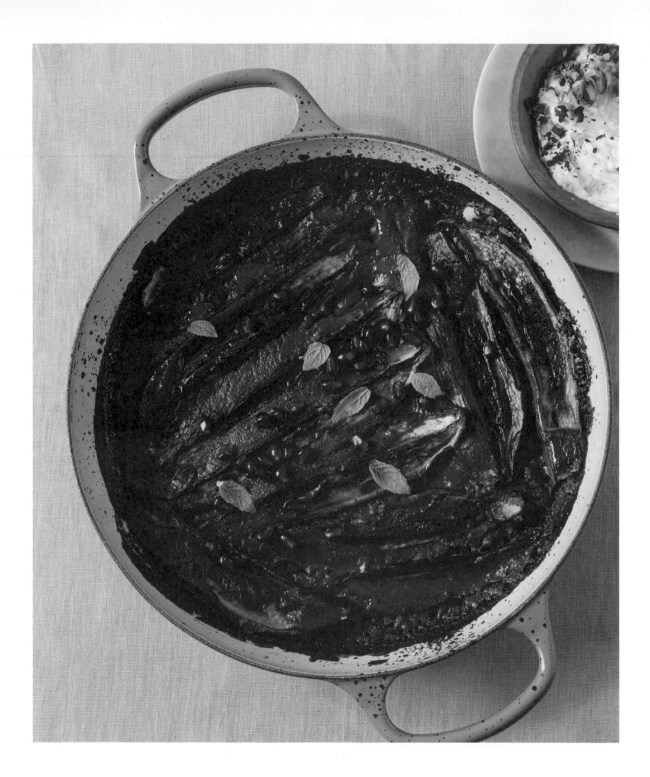

THE GOOD STARCH

Carbohydrates—found in whole grains, beans, starchy and even standard vegetables—are your friend. Carbohydrates mean energy, and every body needs and burns it to function. Where, when, and how much you consume is up to you to become aware of. Slower-release whole grains are excellent for prolonged energy, whereas a starchy vegetable, such as carrot, or a piece of fruit gives a more immediate release of energy. Some people have a bit of starchy carbs at every meal; others prefer to front-load their day with energy. Some still find that their body responds the best with carbs at the end of the day, as a bit of grounding, thus opting for a Runny Egg Bowl at breakfast, a Kale and Preserved Lemon Caesar at lunch, and Gentle Lentils with a tomato toast at dinner. Play around with your carbohydrate intake, with the intention of a more balanced digestive state. Quick tweaks offering immediate improvement have been anywhere from no starch after 4:00 PM, to starting your day in a savory fashion utilizing Gentle Lentils to light your digestive fire, to switching from rice to Healing Congee if emotions and stress are piqued. People all over the world consume grains and starches, often with a staple cultural preparation, sustaining the community in the present and generations prior. I have sought these out in my own adventures and present to you a global tour of rice, bean, and lentil dishes to act as a simple meal, a base, or a side. All are excellent to make a batch of ahead of time, preparing you for an energizing Clean week of whole food opportunities.

MISO BROWN RICE

An excellent refrigerator staple. This rice dish can be reheated as the base of a bowl, as a side, or even, for the adventurous type, fried with an egg for a two-minute meal. During a work hiatus, while finishing my health coaching certification, I would abstain from outsourcing meals to save money and would make batches of this one-pot wonder as the base for many of my meals. I achieved nutrition on a budget every time with very little effort. I like to soak my brown rice to remove the phytic acid, found in the bran of the rice, for easier digestion and absorption of nutrients. The soaking also aids in the cooking process, resulting in a soft brown rice with a consistency that complements the soft sweet potato and miso. Kombu, a variety of seaweed rich in minerals, is an essential component to making the cooking liquid for this rice, as it helps your body digest hearty grains and legumes. A dollop of white miso at the end completes this nutritional powerhouse.

Makes 8 servings

2 cups (360 g) short-grain brown rice

4-inch (10 cm) piece kombu

5½ ounces (150 g) sweet potato
  (about ½ potato)

2 tablespoons sweet white miso paste

Super Seed Blend (page 108),
  optional

1. Rinse the brown rice with water, place in a medium bowl, and cover with 4 cups (960 ml) fresh water. Let stand for 30 minutes.

2. Meanwhile, combine 4 cups (960 ml) water with the kombu in a separate bowl and allow to sit for 30 minutes at room temperature while you peel and dice the sweet potato into ½-inch (13 mm) cubes.

3. Drain the rice, then combine the rice, kombu, and kombu water as well as sweet potato in a rice cooker or 5-quart (5 L) heavy-bottomed, lidded pot.

4. Cook the rice in the rice cooker per the manufacturer's instructions, or in the pot, covered, over medium heat for 30 minutes, until the rice absorbs all the water. Turn off the heat and allow to sit with the lid on for 10 minutes.

5. Remove the lid and remove the kombu. Add the miso paste and fold into the rice.

6. Serve immediately or allow to cool before storing in fridge for up to 5 days until ready to reheat, serving with Super Seed Blend, if desired.

NOTES

I recommend keeping this in the fridge all week for a scoop with this or that, on its own, or added to miso broth with Braised Blue Zone Greens (page 70) to create a quick soup in a pinch.

BLISTERED MISO SWEET POTATOES

My Uncle Robbie taught me to always stay curious, and curious are these potatoes. He loved to learn new techniques and share them with me, blistering potatoes being one of them. I have adapted the technique to sweet potatoes, bringing a Clean Enough perspective to a spud.

He would be rolling his eyes at me right now: *The humble potato isn't good enough for you?* Canadians are *very* attached to their potatoes. This technique gives a nod to blanching potatoes before frying at a high heat to lend a fluffy and ultracrisp texture to the final french fried product. Sweet potatoes are, by nature, moister and softer, but the same technique of boiling and then cooking at a high heat, using a broiler instead of a deep fryer, results in a blistered crispy top that further benefits from a dousing of gut-friendly miso.

Makes 6 to 8 servings

1½ pounds (675 g/4 medium) sweet potatoes or yams, skin on, washed

1 tablespoon plain sesame oil

1½ tablespoons white miso paste

1½ tablespoons hot water

1 tablespoon grated fresh ginger

½ teaspoon fresh lemon juice

¼ teaspoon freshly ground black pepper

Super Seed Blend (page 108), optional

1. Cut each sweet potato in half lengthwise, then in half widthwise. If your potatoes are smaller, simply cut them in half lengthwise.

2. Place the potatoes in a large, heavy-bottomed pot and fill with fresh cold water to cover. Bring to a boil and cook over high heat until fork-tender, about 15 minutes. Drain immediately and allow to cool.

3. Turn on the broiler and place the cooled potatoes, cut side up, on an unlined half sheet pan. Brush the cut sides with the sesame oil and place under the broiler for 15 minutes, or until crisped.

4. Meanwhile, whisk together the miso and hot water in a small bowl to form a thin, opaque paste. Whisk in the ginger and lemon juice.

5. When the potatoes are done, immediately brush with the miso mixture and grind fresh pepper over the top. Sprinkle with Super Seed Blend, if using. Serve immediately.

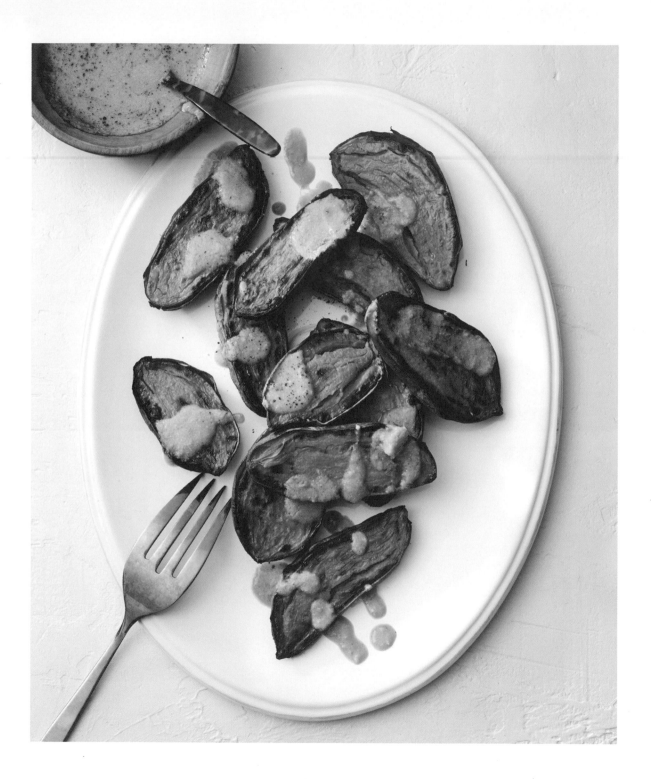

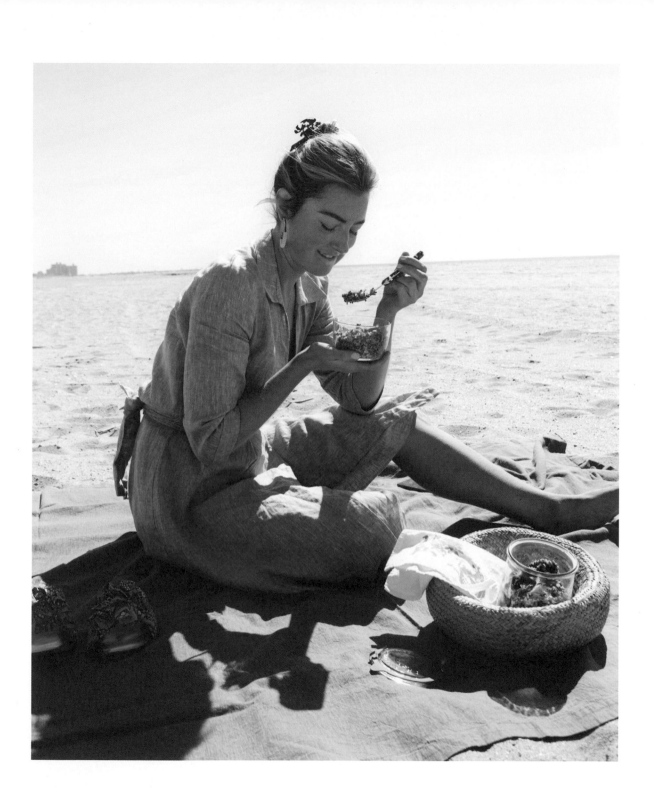

THE GOOD STARCH

PERUVIAN QUINOA

Welcome to Mancora, a fishing village that appeals to surfers and yogis alike, tucked away in northwestern Peru. There, a bite of local fish with dressed quinoa is a lunch staple. Quinoa has sustained the people of Peru for centuries: a high-protein energy source that has carried people on the Inca trail, eventually making its way to the United States as a new superfood. Disclaimer: It is actually a seed, not a grain, pointing to its complete protein content, meaning its complete amino acid profile. While traveling and during my stay there I may have been doing more downward dogs and napping than hiking, yet I still had my fill of this tastily prepared grain that fueled me through twice-daily treetop sun salutations.

Makes 6 servings

1 tablespoon extra virgin olive oil

1 small red onion, diced

1 garlic clove, peeled and minced

3 cups (720 ml) unsalted organic vegetable stock

1½ cups (225 g) uncooked quinoa

1 avocado

1 cup (60 g) fresh parsley leaves, chopped

2 tablespoons fresh lemon juice

½ teaspoon Himalayan pink salt

¼ teaspoon freshly ground black pepper

1. Heat a medium pot and add the olive oil. Sauté the onion and garlic until translucent, about 5 minutes. Add the vegetable stock and bring to a simmer.

2. Whisk in the quinoa, cover, and cook for 15 minutes. The quinoa is finished when it becomes translucent, with a little tail detaching from the seed. Turn off the heat and keep the pot covered.

3. Peel and pit the avocado, place in a large bowl, and mash into a chunky puree. Fold in the parsley and lemon juice along with the salt and pepper.

4. Fluff the quinoa and fold into the avocado mash. Serve immediately at room temperature or cold.

___

NOTES

This is an excellent base to a bowl with a soft-boiled egg on top (page 27) and dressed greens.

Grab a few leftover butter lettuce leaves from the Radish Peas Parmesan salad (page 52) and fill with this quinoa for a mini wrap.

EASTERN MEDICINE HEALTH RICE

My visits to Seoul always included this rice. I would eat it for breakfast, lunch, and sometimes dinner. The rice first attracted me with its translated hotel description of being a "health" rice. In a state of jet lag and not feeling my best, which usually accompanied at least a portion of my overseas travel, this rice gave me solace. My body felt good, and I knew I was making a positive choice for myself. I have worked on this rice to make it multistep yet achievable, resulting in a bright purple pot of nourishment that can be enjoyed a multitude of ways. I love using it as the base of my at-home Bibimbap (page 88), but simply mixing in some leafy greens is a just-as-satisfying pairing.

Makes 8 to 10 servings

½ cup (90 g) dried adzuki red or kidney beans

½ cup (90 g) dried black beans

½ cup (90 g) uncooked brown rice

1 cup (185 g) uncooked black rice

½ cup (90 g) short-grain white rice

1 cup (200 g) uncooked millet

2 teaspoons Himalayan pink salt

1 cup (145 g) chestnuts, roasted whole and peeled, then roughly chopped

1. Combine the red and black beans in the same large pot, cover with water, bring to a boil, and turn off the heat. Allow them to sit for 1 hour before draining and using in the recipe.

2. At the 30-minute point of quick-soaking the beans, place the rice (brown, black, and white) and millet in medium bowl, cover with fresh water, and let soak for 30 minutes.

3. Drain the quick-soaked beans and rice and place in a large, lidded pot with 10 cups (2.4 L) water, salt, and the chopped chestnuts.

4. Bring to a simmer and cook, uncovered, for 30 minutes over medium-high heat.

5. Lower the heat and cook, covered, for 15 minutes, being careful to not burn the rice or grains on the bottom of the pot.

6. Turn off the heat and allow the rice to sit, covered, for another 15 minutes.

7. Fluff and serve immediately or allow to cool and then store in the fridge until ready to reheat.

NOTES

Millet is a petite grain that looks like couscous when it is raw. It is gluten-free and full of fiber and minerals, keeping most people's digestive tract healthy and blood sugar stabilized.

Most rice is cooked and steamed, but this rice includes beans, which need more liquid to cook. Be sure to check the bottom of the pot so that the rice does not burn as the beans are cooking.

BIBIMBAP

Traditionally served in a piping hot stone bowl, bibimbap is a cinch to make at home. I will often order this when eating out with friends at a Korean restaurant or while traveling, as it is the easiest way to eat Clean and be in control of what ingredients you are putting in your body. (I am sensitive to too many extra sauces that are often full of sugar and preservatives, and while I am of the Clean Enough mentality, sometimes it is worth it, but other times I do not want to risk a headache from my dinner!) Bibimbap is easily modified both at home and in a restaurant, where you can focus on healthful rice and fresh vegetables on top. Don't forget the Kraut (page 112), our Clean take on kimchi, an excellent probiotic.

Makes 4 servings

1 tablespoon extra virgin olive oil

4 cups (640 g) Eastern Medicine Health Rice (page 87)

4 pasture-raised eggs

2 cups (240 g) Sesame Cucumber Salad (page 68)

1⅓ cups (150 g) Kraut (page 112)

1 zucchini (5½ ounces/150 g)

2 tablespoons Rooster Sauce (page 116) or more as desired

1 cup (40 g) fresh cilantro leaves, chopped

OPTIONAL

1 batch Midnight Carrots (page 78)

1 batch Braised Blue Zone Greens (page 70)

1 batch Eat the Rainbow Salad (page 62)

1. Heat 2 teaspoons of the olive oil in a cast-iron skillet. Add the rice to reheat and slightly fry, cooking for 5 minutes. Divide the rice among four bowls.

2. Lightly wipe out the skillet and heat the remaining teaspoon of oil. Cook the eggs sunny-side up, covered to circulate the heat (see Runny Egg Bowl, page 27–28).

3. Meanwhile, place the cucumber salad and sauerkraut on top of the rice.

4. Grate the zucchini, using a boxed grater, or peel into long ribbons. Place on top of the rice, next to the cucumber.

5. Place a cooked egg on top of each rice bowl and drizzle each bowl with 1½ teaspoons of the Rooster Sauce. Sprinkle with chopped cilantro and serve immediately. Top with Midnight Carrots, Braised Blue Zone Greens, or Eat the Rainbow Salad, if using.

NOTES

You can switch up the vegetable toppings to your liking. Some vegetables, such as the carrots, can be added cooked and cooled, whereas others will benefit from reheating before being added to the top of the rice bowl.

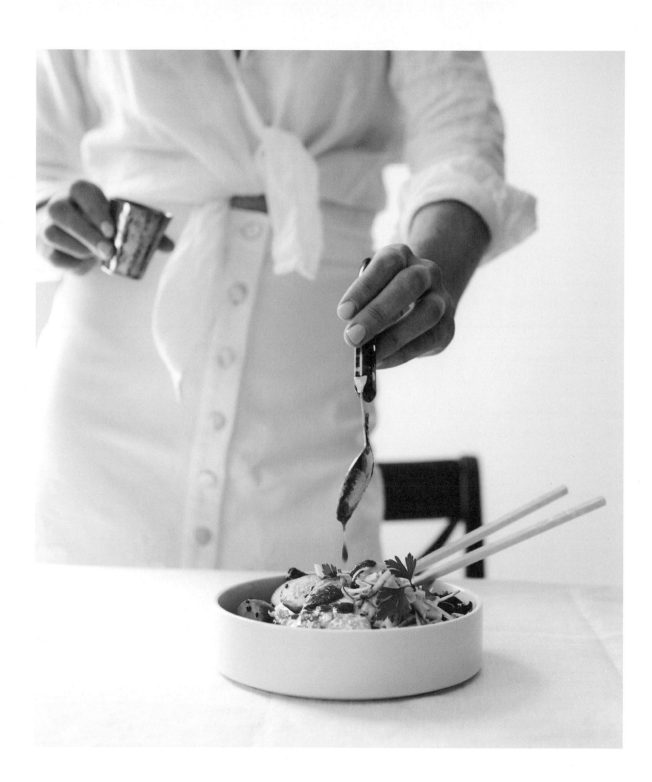

GENTLE LENTILS

Lentils are easy to make, easy on your digestion, and all around a loving way to feed yourself and others. Do not be afraid of the plethora of spices; these are pantry staples that further light your digestive fire in this dish. This is a hybrid of Indian *kitchari* and a favorite Middle Eastern lentil dish (made with zucchini instead of potato)—ancient dishes that will be relevant as long as we have stomachs and emotions to turn them. Asking someone what they were given when they were not well is a fascinating high-mileage question. Whether they were suffering from the flu, an upset stomach, a bad day at school, a heartbreak; people often remember that meals shared during such times were warming, nourishing, and grounding—just like these gentle lentils, which not only deliver a great source of protein, but are the easiest legume to digest even without the addition of all the healing spices.

Makes 6 servings

1 tablespoon extra virgin olive oil

1 small yellow onion, diced into ¼-inch (6 mm) pieces

1 zucchini (5½ ounces/150 g), diced into ¼-inch (6 mm) pieces

1 teaspoon fennel seeds

1 teaspoon ground coriander

1 teaspoon ground mustard seeds

1 teaspoon ground turmeric

1 teaspoon paprika

½ teaspoon dried oregano

½ teaspoon freshly ground black pepper

½ teaspoon ground cumin

1½ cups (360 ml) unsalted organic vegetable stock

2 cups (360 g) dried red lentils

1 teaspoon Himalayan pink salt

1. Heat the olive oil in a heavy-bottomed, lidded pot over medium heat and add the onion. Sauté until translucent, 5 minutes. Add the zucchini and continue to sauté for 5 minutes.

2. Meanwhile, place all the spices and herbs in a small, dry skillet and toast slightly over medium heat for about 3 minutes.

3. Add the spice mixture to the onion mixture along with the vegetable stock, lentils, and 2½ cups (600 ml) water. Simmer, covered, for 20 minutes, then turn off the heat and fold in the salt.

4. Serve immediately or allow to cool and then store in the fridge until ready to reheat, adding a few tablespoons of water, as it becomes very thick when cold.

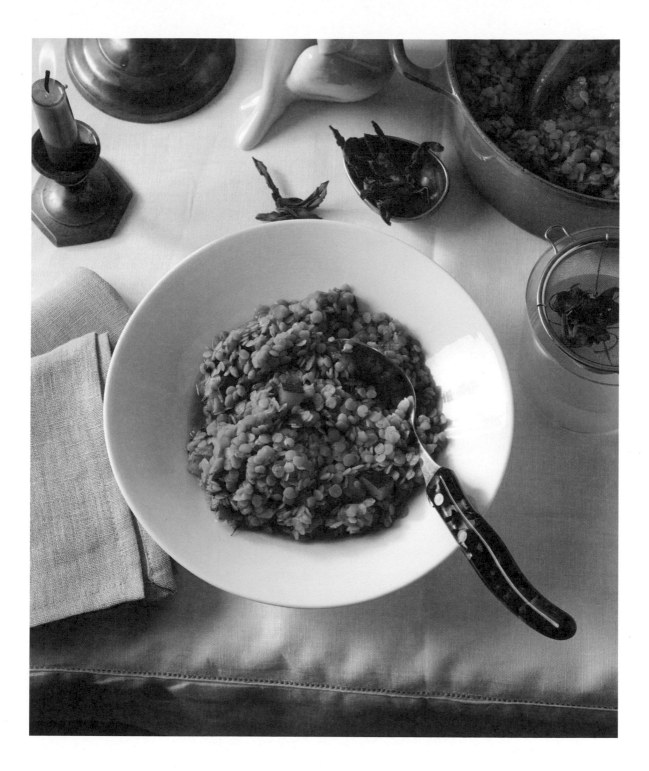

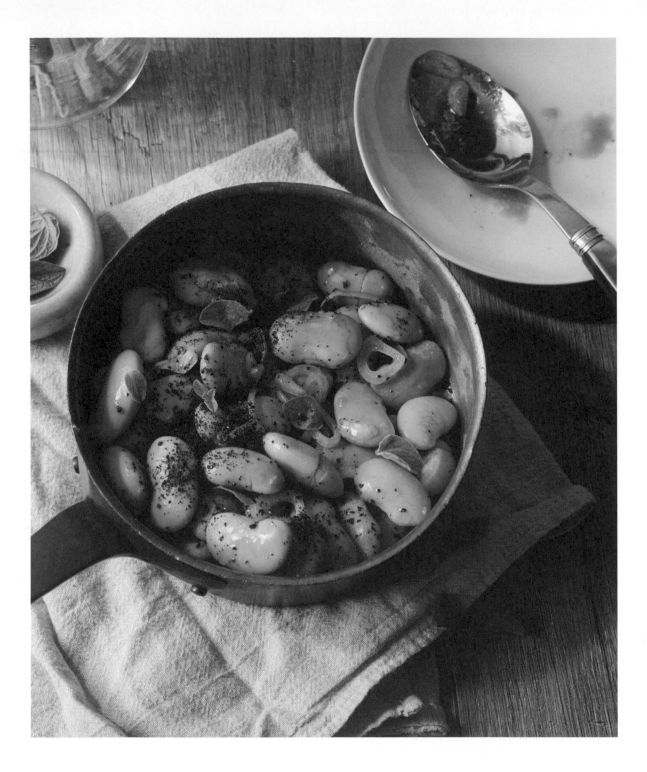

SUMAC AND OREGANO GIGANTE BEANS

I say "yigante", you say "gigante"—either way, these broad white beans are so delicious. As they are a staple in Greek and Italian cuisines, I am a fan of mixing it up by adding trusty sour sumac and pungent fresh oregano. Canned gigante beans are usually found in the legume aisle, imported from Italy, or already macerated at the serve-yourself olive bar in most grocery stores, but soaking and cooking them yourself is simple and allows you to have these beans on hand at any moment. The beans are protein and fiber-rich, with a host of antioxidants coming from the sumac and immunity-boosting, antimicrobial oregano to round out this very simple recipe.

Makes 4 servings

2 cups (400 g) dried gigante beans
  (see Notes)

1 tablespoon extra virgin olive oil

1 shallot, sliced thinly

1 garlic clove, minced

¼ teaspoon Himalayan pink salt

1 teaspoon sumac

1 heaping tablespoon fresh oregano
  leaves, roughly chopped

2 tablespoons red wine vinegar

1. Place the gigante beans in 10 cups (2.4 L) fresh water and bring to a boil, immediately turn off the heat, and let soak for 1 hour.

2. Drain the beans, place in a large, lidded pot, and cover with fresh water. Bring to a boil and cook, covered, for about 50 minutes to cook thoroughly.

3. Allow the beans to sit, covered, in their cooking liquid until ready to use, then drain 2 cups (340 g) of the cooked beans and rinse with cool water. Refrigerate any remaining beans in their cooking liquid.

4. Heat the olive oil in a large sauté pan over medium heat, add the shallot and garlic, and sauté until translucent, 5 minutes.

5. Increase the heat to medium-high and add the gigante beans. Sauté to caramelize slightly, then add the salt, sumac, and chopped oregano to the pan. Toss to heat through.

6. Turn off the heat and add the vinegar. Serve immediately.

NOTES

You will have leftover cooked gigante beans. If you cook a batch of gigante beans ahead of time, store them in the fridge in their unsalted cooking liquid until ready to drain and sauté in the recipe. Use leftover beans to add to salads and soups or to top toasts for a hearty, protein-rich, and complex carbohydrate addition.

These beans also make an excellent puree. Simply add the finished recipe to a food processor and pulse until smooth. Serve with Midnight Carrots (page 78), Charred Pumpkin Seed Broccolini (page 72), fresh radishes, or other vegetables to dip. Alternatively, pile the Kale and Preserved Lemon Caesar (page 48) on top of the puree to serve.

SPINACH RICE

I have dreams about this rice, a Greek staple found in any neighborhood restaurant and the ultimate accompaniment to gigante beans for a complete supper. The rice soaks up the tomato liquid for the most flavorful dish that you can fathom. Sautéed spinach with a whisper of nutmeg rounds everything out. Iron, lycopene, grains for energy, nothing more to say.

Makes 4 to 6 servings

8 ounces (225 g) fresh baby spinach

1 tablespoon extra virgin olive oil

1 small yellow onion, minced

1 garlic clove, minced

1 pound (450 g) organic tomatoes, peeled and crushed

½ cup (85 g) uncooked long-grain basmati rice, rinsed

¼ teaspoon lemon zest

2 teaspoons fresh lemon juice

½ teaspoon Himalayan pink salt

¼ teaspoon freshly ground black pepper

¼ teaspoon paprika

⅛ teaspoon freshly grated nutmeg

1 cup (240 ml) unsalted organic vegetable stock

1. Place a tablespoon of water in a skillet over medium-high heat and add the spinach to just wilt. Remove the spinach from the heat, squeeze out the bitter liquid, and set the spinach aside.

2. Heat the oil in a heavy-bottomed, lidded pot over medium heat and add the minced onion and garlic. Cook until translucent, about 10 minutes. Add the tomatoes and simmer for 5 minutes.

3. Add the rice, lemon zest and juice, salt, pepper, paprika, and nutmeg. Stir to combine.

4. Add the vegetable stock and spinach. Simmer, covered, for 30 minutes.

5. Serve immediately or allow to cool and then store in the fridge until ready to reheat.

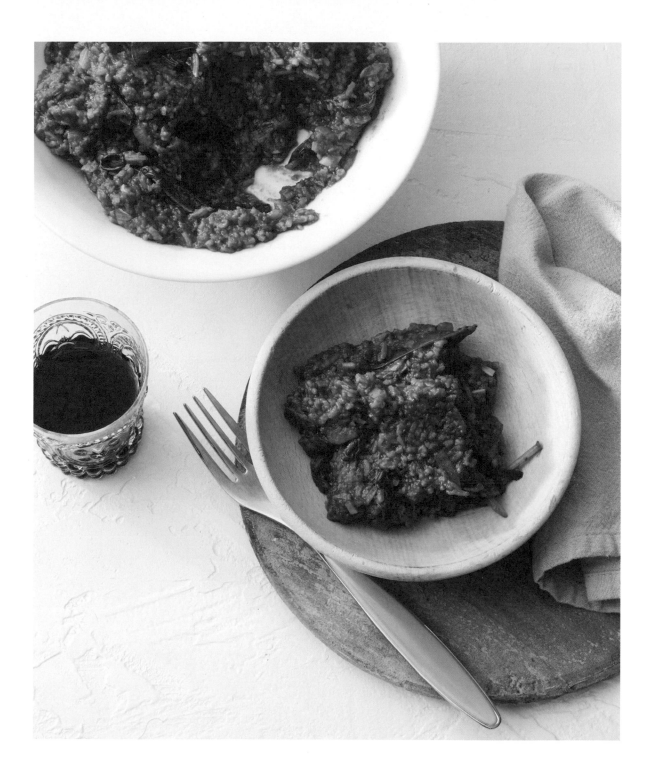

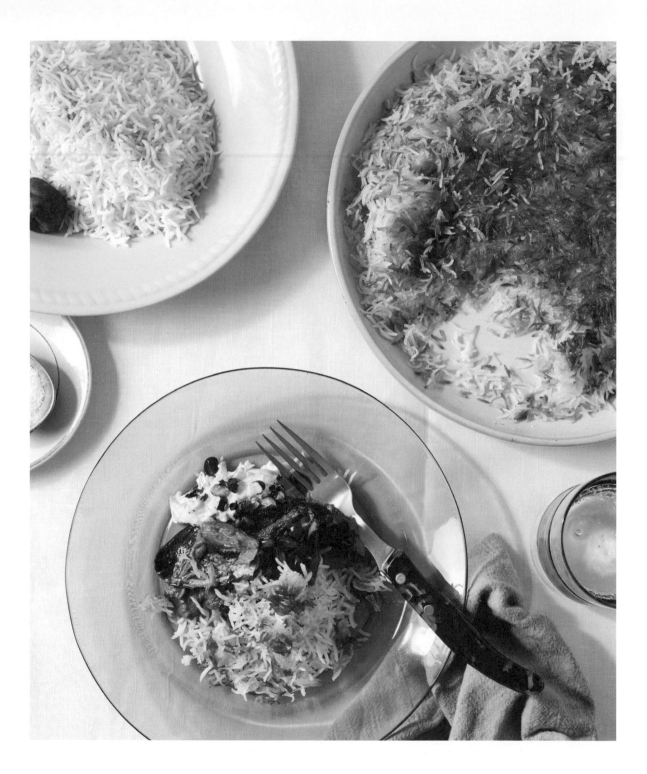

COCONUT OIL CRISPY RICE

This Persian rice is not any old rice. Unlike with the Miso Brown Rice, the cooking process here is mindful and delicate. The crispy layer is the ultimate treat in this recipe. Known as *tah dig*, it forms during the steaming of the basmati rice on the bottom of the pot. A good tah dig is judged by its even, golden-brown crust as well as its easy release from the bottom of the pot. You essentially scoop out the steamed rice and then turn the pot upside down in hopes that the tah dig pops out fully intact onto a plate. Saffron threads, the most luxurious spice on earth, add a touch of color and earthiness to the finished rice.

Makes 10 servings

3 cups (540 g) uncooked basmati rice

3 tablespoons unrefined coconut oil

1 Persian lime (or ½ regular lime)

½ teaspoon Himalayan pink salt

Pinch of saffron threads

1. Rinse the rice with fresh running water three times, or until the water runs clear. Place the rice in a bowl, cover with cold water, and allow to sit at room temperature for 30 minutes. Meanwhile, bring a large pot of water to a boil.

2. Add the rinsed rice to the boiling water and cook for 6 minutes, or until the grains begin to dance at the top of the pot. Immediately drain the rice and rinse with cold water, then set aside.

3. Melt the coconut oil in the bottom of a large, lidded pot. Place a 2-inch (5 cm) layer of rice carefully on the bottom of the pot, packing it down slightly and sprinkling with salt. Spoon the remaining rice into the center of the pot, creating a pile of rice. Tuck the Persian lime inside the rice pile.

4. Wrap the lid of the pot with a tea towel and place on the pot. Reduce the heat to low and steam the rice for about 40 minutes, until the rice is steamed and fluffy and the bottom of the pot has crisped and is golden brown. Until you get used to this process you can peek at the edge with a spoon to see how it is doing after 30 or 35 minutes.

5. Carefully scoop the steamed rice out onto a plate, leaving the bottom packed-down rice intact. Then, using a plate the diameter of the pot, place the plate on top of the pot and flip the pot over, releasing the tah dig from the bottom of the pot.

6. Grind the saffron thread with a mortar and pestle and add a tablespoon of water to make a saffron slurry. Spoon this over the finished rice. Serve the tah dig next to the rice along with Tzatziki or plain Labne (page 109).

SOUP'S ON

My favorite thing to order in a foreign country is the local soup. This is a gentle way for me to deal with jet lag and taste the flavors and the spices of the region in their glory, along with sampling a local approach to healing, feeding groups affordably, and utilizing everything that is available, even scraps. Bottom line, I also just love soup, so I know I won't be disappointed. Soup is the original smoothie: a savory blend packed with vitamins, minerals, healthy fats, protein, and useful carbohydrates. It supports your system and can be a great digestive reset, enjoyed in place of hearty raw salads in the evening, for instance, easing your body into a resting state. Soups nourish, heal while also allowing your body to direct its energy to balance rather than breaking down a meal. They are a great act of self-care during weeks when you're rattled with exhaustion from environmental or hormonal factors. They also instantly warm you up, whether it be on a ski slope or in ski socks in your living room. Even when home in New York, I often walk around with a coffee cup of soup, a little secret of mine when I need to keep something warm in my body that's a bit more substantial than tea, and when it is not time for a meal.

As with many Clean foods, making your own gives you full range of control of the sugar and salt content. Soups can have a sneaky ability to fulfill over half of your daily recommendation for sodium in one serving when purchased on the run. By making your own, adjusting the seasoning to taste as you go, using high-quality electrolyte-balancing Himalayan pink salt and pungent fresh herbs and spices, you will not run into the swollen-fingers scenario in the middle of the night. These soups all contain their own unique nutrient punch, from bright orange squash to deep red beets, to herbaceous coconut, anti-inflammatory congee, and fresh juicy tomato. A final secret? I often ladle soup straight over a bowl of raw or steamed greens; soup's on!

FERMENTED GARLIC AND SQUASH SOUP

I have never met Mrs. Hiroshi, yet I adore her soup. The directions were given to me on an index card, her name written across the top with the instructions describing a Clean Enough and satisfying soup of vitamin-rich squash and pungent thyme. Thus, inspiring me to layer in the sweet flavor of fermented black garlic, lending a backdrop of "hmm, what is it?" to the puree. Roasting the squash prior to adding it to the cooking liquid brings out its natural sweetness, without having to add sugar, which surprisingly can be found in many off-the-shelf soups. Squash is a go-to for many, as it seems to be a vegetable that when cooked truly supports digestion and is agreeable to most regardless of their dietary needs.

Makes 6 servings

3 pounds (1.4 kg) butternut or kabocha squash, peeled, seeded, and cubed (8 cups)

3 tablespoons extra virgin olive oil

1 large Vidalia onion, diced (1½ cups/240 g)

¾ teaspoon peeled and minced fermented black garlic (about ¾ large clove)

5 thyme sprigs

2 cups (480 ml) filtered water

1 cup (240 ml) unsalted organic vegetable stock

2 tablespoons unfiltered cider vinegar

2 teaspoons Himalayan pink salt

½ teaspoon freshly ground black pepper, plus more for sprinkling

¼ teaspoon crushed red pepper flakes

5 ounces (145 g) cooked and peeled chestnuts, chopped (1 cup)

¼ teaspoon freshly grated nutmeg

¼ teaspoon Maldon sea salt flakes

Lemon wedges

Super Seed Blend (page 108), optional

1. Preheat the oven to 400°F (200°C). Place the cubed squash on an unlined half sheet pan and toss with 1 tablespoon of the olive oil. Place in the oven to roast for 30 minutes, tossing the squash halfway through to roast evenly.

2. Heat 1 tablespoon of the olive oil in a heavy-bottomed pot over medium-low heat and add the onion, black garlic, and thyme. Sauté for 20 minutes to slowly caramelize the onion.

3. Add the water, vegetable stock, vinegar, and squash to the onion mixture. Bring to a simmer and cook for 15 minutes. Remove the thyme sprigs and stir in the pink salt, black pepper, and crushed red pepper.

4. Transfer the soup to a high-powered blender or use an immersion stick blender and puree until ultrasmooth.

5. Heat the final tablespoon of olive oil in a sauté pan over medium-high heat and add the chestnuts. Brown the chestnuts, about 4 minutes, then season with the nutmeg and sea salt.

6. Serve the soup with freshly ground black pepper, wedges of lemon, and the pan-crisped chestnuts along with Super Seed Blend, if using.

TOMATO BLITZ

A little goes a long way with the onion and garlic in this fresh tomato soup. The first time I made it, I created a monster that stank up the house, car, fridge, and crowd. The memory of doing laps around a parking garage to air out the car makes me laugh out loud every time I think of it. Use juicy heirloom beefsteak tomatoes for the brightest flavor and antioxidant-rich lycopene, and top with toasted almonds, which lend a great texture and flavor along with vitamin E, fiber, and protein.

Makes 4 to 5 servings

½ small red onion

½ garlic clove, peeled

2 pounds (900 g) heirloom tomatoes

1 ounce (25 g) fresh fennel bulb, roughly chopped, fronds reserved for garnish

1 scallion, chopped

½ cup (75 g) whole almonds, toasted

¼ cup (60 ml) extra virgin olive oil

3 tablespoons red wine vinegar

2 teaspoons freshly ground black pepper

1½ teaspoons Himalayan pink salt

1 teaspoon fresh lemon juice

2 teaspoons basil leaf chiffonade (cut into ribbons)

3½ ounces (100 g) Persian cucumber, diced (⅔ cup)

1 batch Tzatziki (page 109)

1. Slice the red onion and garlic and place in a bowl of cold fresh water for 15 minutes.

2. Roughly chop the tomatoes, discarding the white core.

3. Place the drained red onion and garlic, tomatoes, fennel, chopped scallion, and toasted almonds in a high-powered blender. Blend on high speed until smooth, about 1 minute.

4. Season with the olive oil, vinegar, pepper, salt, and lemon juice. Blend to combine, about 15 seconds. Add the basil and blend briefly, about 5 seconds, to incorporate the basil flavor.

5. Stir in the diced cucumber and chill in the fridge for an hour before serving.

6. Top with Tzatziki and leftover fennel fronds from the bulb.

VELVET BEET

I have a thing for borscht, a traditional Russian or Ukrainian beet soup that has more iterations than apple pie. I like my borscht with cabbage and pureed until smooth and creamy with a heavy dusting of poppy seeds and fresh dill. If borscht is on the menu, I am sure to order it, especially when in Russia. Beet is a blood purifier, rich in fiber and antioxidants.

Makes 6 to 8 servings

1 pound (450 g) beets, peeled and cubed

2 tablespoons extra virgin olive oil

1 small yellow onion, diced

1 large carrot, diced

2 celery stalks, diced

1 bunch fresh dill, chopped

1½ teaspoons blue poppy seeds, plus more for sprinkling

½ teaspoon ground coriander

¼ teaspoon ground cumin

5 ounces (2 cups/140 g) shredded green cabbage

6 cups (1.4 L) filtered water

1 heaping tablespoon organic tomato paste

1 tablespoon cider vinegar

2½ teaspoons Himalayan pink salt

1 teaspoon freshly ground black pepper

2 tablespoons (60 g) Kraut (page 112) with its juice

2 teaspoons fresh lemon juice

1 batch Tzatziki (page 109)

6 to 8 thin slices dark rye bread, each about 1 cm thick, toasted

Goat's milk butter

1. Preheat the oven to 400°F (200°C). Place the cubed beets on a half sheet pan, toss with 1 tablespoon of the olive oil, and roast in the oven for 30 to 40 minutes, until tender.

2. Heat the remaining tablespoon of oil in a large pot and add the onion, carrot, celery, and all except 2 tablespoons of the dill. Sauté over medium heat for 10 minutes.

3. Add 1 teaspoon of the poppy seeds, the coriander, and cumin to the onion mixture, followed by the roasted beets and raw cabbage. Sauté over medium-high heat for 5 minutes.

4. Add the water, tomato paste, vinegar, 2 teaspoons of the salt, and ½ teaspoon of the pepper. Simmer for 30 minutes.

5. Remove from the heat and add the 2 tablespoons of reserved fresh dill along with the Kraut and its juice.

6. Transfer to a high-powered blender and blend until smooth.

7. Season with the lemon juice and remaining the ½ teaspoon each of the poppy seeds, salt, and black pepper.

8. Serve with Tzatziki and rye bread toasted and smeared with goat's milk butter and poppy seeds.

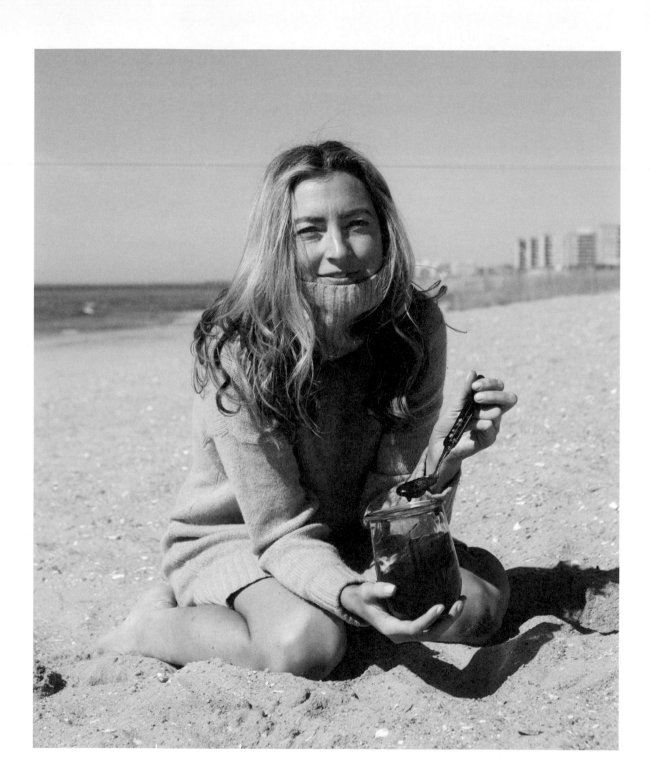

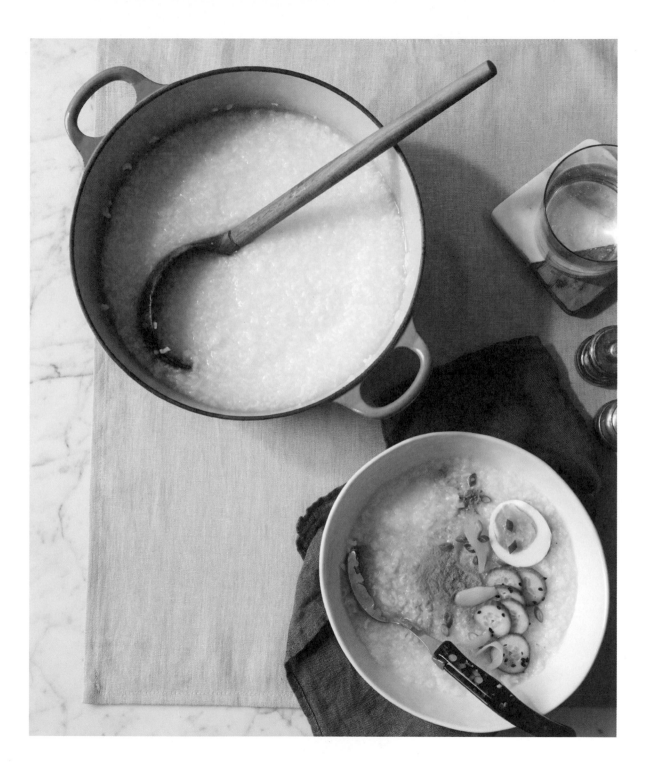

HEALING CONGEE

Beijing. Not the city center, but the outskirts. Something is amiss. I am there solo and judgmental of myself for not feeling well. I must be faking it; buck up, it's jet lag. Or it is the pollution? The index says that it is at a toxic level; I can't go outside as it's giving me a headache. I use my internet portal, as the standard internet is blocked, to reach out to friends in the States; they say I must be tired. Fast-forward, and I'm the sickest I have been so far in my life in a place that is only contributing to my ailment. I still remember making the hotel general manager walk me across the street to the twenty-four-hour makeshift pharmacy in the middle of the night to get something, anything over-the-counter remotely described as "medicine."

Herein lies the very dramatic beginnings of my love affair with congee. This rice porridge nursed me back to life. Congee is simple: rice cooked slowly, which breaks down the grain for soothing and easy digestion. Congee can be eaten in a savory or naturally sweet context—topped with a runny egg, cinnamon, turmeric, pickled ginger, honey, you name it—and it's very soothing in all iterations. I personally prefer it plain and simple.

Makes 4 servings

12 cups (2.9 L) filtered water

⅔ cup (130 g) short-grain white rice

½ teaspoon Himalayan pink salt

TOPPINGS

1 runny egg (page 27–28), any variety

Pickled ginger

Rooster Sauce (page 116)

Ground turmeric

Sliced scallion

Super Seed Blend (page 108),
  optional

or

Ground cinnamon

Ground turmeric

Raw honey

1. Combine the water, rice, and salt in a large heavy-bottomed, lidded saucepan. Bring to a simmer and cook for 1½ to 2 hours, whisking three times spaced evenly along the cooking process, until the rice is cooked down and porridge-like.

2. To serve, ladle the congee into a bowl and top with a runny egg, pickled ginger, Rooster Sauce, turmeric, and scallion along with Super Seed Blend, if using. Or, for a sweet porridge option, dust with cinnamon and turmeric and drizzle with honey.

3. Congee can be cooled and stored in the fridge for reheating.

COSTA RICAN COCONUT SOUP

A hot summer night after a day at the beach is complete with a shallow bowl of rich, flavorful, yet Clean Enough soup. Follow it by an evening stroll and a nine o'clock bedtime and that right there is a life well lived. I discovered this type of soup in Nosara, Costa Rica, where, as in many hot climates, hot soup is enjoyed and used as a temperature regulator. Try it the next time you have a sweaty August evening, changing it up to have a hot yet light soup. This soup can be made in a flash, so I prefer to not make it ahead; rather, I toss it together and sit down in a moment to pure coconut bliss. The tofu is optional and adds an additional layer of protein and nutrition to this fresh broth.

Makes 6 servings

¼ cup (60 g) unrefined coconut oil

6 scallions (green and white parts separated), sliced thinly

1 pound (450 g) baby portobello mushrooms, sliced (3 cups)

12½ ounces (375 g) carrots, grated (3 cups)

About 11 ounces (300 g) firm tofu, drained and cubed, optional

¾ cup (30 g) cilantro leaves, chopped

4½ cups (1.1 L) organic coconut milk (about three 13.5-ounce/400 ml cans)

2¼ cups (540 ml) unsalted organic vegetable stock

¼ cup (60 g) Rooster Sauce (page 116)

3 tablespoons (45 ml) Bragg Liquid Aminos

¼ cup + 2 tablespoons (90 ml) fresh lime juice (from about 3 limes)

5 ounces (140 g) radishes, sliced into matchsticks (1 cup)

¾ cup (30 g) fresh basil leaves, julienned

¾ cup (70 g) fresh mint leaves

1. Heat the coconut oil in a heavy-bottomed pot over medium-high heat and add the chopped white scallion. Sauté for 3 minutes. Add the sliced mushrooms and sauté over high heat until tender, 4 to 5 minutes.

2. Add the carrots, tofu (if using), cilantro, and chopped green scallion. Sauté for 2 minutes.

3. Add the coconut milk, vegetable stock, Rooster Sauce, and liquid aminos. Bring to a simmer and cook for 5 minutes, then remove from the heat and season the soup with the lime juice.

4. Serve the soup with the radishes, basil, and mint piled on top.

CLEAN PANTRY

Here you'll find everything you need to know to whip up a quick sauce, dip, or spread as well as the essentials to kick up a harmony bowl, toasts, salad, and the like. Pantry items can change mealtime in an instant. Picky eaters no longer dampen dinner when you offer a spread of condiments, allowing customization for every taste. The pantry items are also great recipes to master, as they offer room for flexibility and creativity. Understanding the basic framework for a pesto and the technique that you prefer to utilize to prepare it gives you freedom to play with herbs, nuts, spices, citrus, and infused oils. Pantry items often are components of a dish or a finishing tool, meaning they come with a high concentration of flavor and function. A small portion of Rose Harissa offers a host of antimicrobial spices, while Guacamole gives you an instant brain boost while acting as a perfect save to your casual hosting duties or nachos craving. Mastering a wide range of dressings for greens will keep your salad game strong, showing you just how easy it is to make your own. As these are all fresh pantry items, they will help you slowly build your physical pantry of spices, vinegars, oils, nuts, and seeds. As you work through the recipes you will be able to discover your favorite tahini paste, miso, extra virgin olive oil, or blend of za'atar. Learning how to make your own basic fermented products will greatly improve your digestive health—this I wholeheartedly promise. By creating something as simple yet seemingly daunting as Kraut, hopefully you will keep it on hand and have a bit with every meal, feeding your gut with the good stuff so that you can digest and live better. Reference this section often as you work through Clean. You are well on your way to Enough.

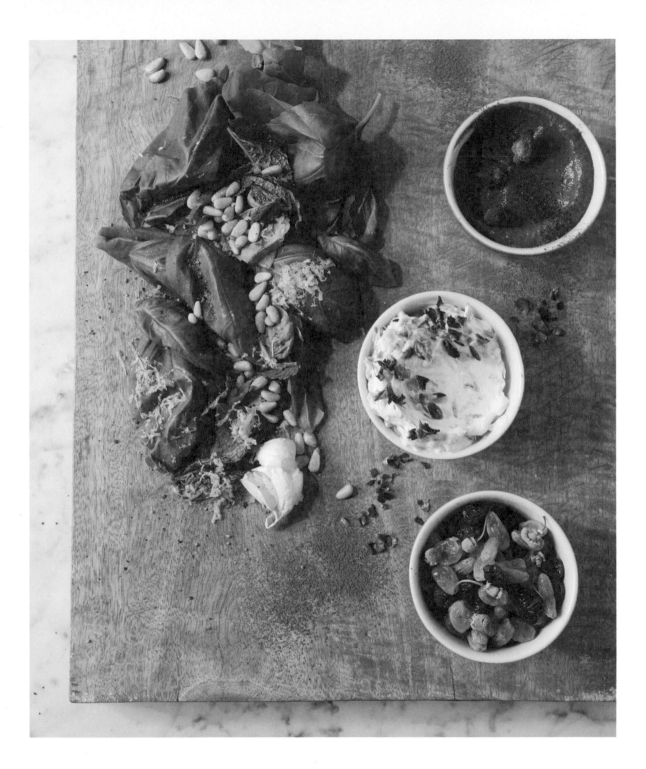

SUPER SEED BLEND

A Clean Enough staple, with anti-inflammatory turmeric activated with black pepper and balanced with Himalayan pink salt. With the healthy fat and protein from hemp, flax, sesame, and pumpkin seeds, this is something to definitely keep on hand for whenever.

Makes 1 cup (150 g)

¼ cup (16 g) raw pumpkin seeds

3 tablespoons ground turmeric

3 tablespoons raw hemp seeds

2 tablespoons flaxseeds

2 tablespoons freshly ground black pepper

2 tablespoons sesame seeds

1 tablespoon Himalayan pink salt

1. Combine all the ingredients in a food processor and pulse until the pumpkin seeds have become roughly ground.

2. Store in an airtight container in the fridge or at room temperature for up 2 weeks.

NOTE

I like to store my super seeds in a shaker with large holes, for easy seasoning.

MISO DRESSING

This dressing is not tied to a specific main dish; however, it is a secret underneath the Avocado Guacamole Toast (page 38) as well as an alternative dressing for the Sesame Cucumber Salad (page 68). I am a huge fan of this as a dip with the Midnight Carrots (page 78).

Makes 2 cups (480 ml)

1 cup + 2 tablespoons (270 ml) filtered water

½ cup (75 g) raw cashews

¼ cup (65 g) organic white miso paste

2 tablespoons + 1 teaspoon fresh lemon juice

2 tablespoons + 1 teaspoon Rooster Sauce (page 116)

1 teaspoon dried mushroom powder

1 teaspoon sliced scallion (white part only)

½ teaspoon black garlic

½ teaspoon Himalayan pink salt

1 tablespoon toasted sesame oil

1 tablespoon thinly sliced scallion (green part only)

1. Combine the water and cashews in a high-powered blender and blend on high speed for 1 minute.

2. Add the miso, lemon juice, Rooster Sauce, mushroom powder, white scallion, black garlic, and salt. Blend on high speed, scraping down, for 1 minute.

3. Transfer to a serving bowl and fold in the thinly sliced green scallion. Use immediately or store in the fridge for up to 2 days.

LABNE + TZATZIKI

What's better than a cucumber yogurt sauce? A cucumber yogurt sauce made with DIY Labne instead of yogurt. The grated cucumber and rose water loosen the thick and rich Labne, bringing a refreshing flavor to the condiment that can be used in a wide array of applications. From soups, salads, toasts, and bowls to hors d'oeuvres, use your imagination with this recipe.

Makes 1 cup Tzatziki (225 g)

LABNE

2 cups (450 g) low- or full-fat organic plain Greek yogurt

TZATZIKI

2 heaping tablespoons finely grated Persian cucumber

2 teaspoons finely chopped fresh mint

¼ teaspoon grated lemon zest

1 teaspoon fresh lemon juice

½ teaspoon rose water (Mymouné brand preferred)

¼ teaspoon grated garlic, microplane grated

1 teaspoon chopped pistachios

1 teaspoon food-grade fresh rose petals, crushed

1. To make the Labne: Place the yogurt in cheesecloth or a cold brew or nut milk bag. Hang over a bowl to catch the liquid and place in the fridge for 12 hours. The longer you let the yogurt strain, the thicker it becomes. (For ultrastrained yogurt, hang for 16 hours.) Store your Labne in a glass jar, refrigerated, for up to 2 weeks.

2. To make the Tzatziki: Fold together ½ cup (115 g) of the Labne, the cucumber, mint, lemon zest and juice, rose water, and garlic in a small bowl.

3. Transfer to a small dish and sprinkle the top with the pistachios and rose petals. Serve immediately.

NOTES

You will have leftover Labne. Use it as a spread for the Longevity Mushroom Toast (page 39), or as a thicker, more protein-rich substitute for yogurt in the Harmony Bowls (page 21). Serve atop any grains or add a dollop to your smoothies for a creamy touch.

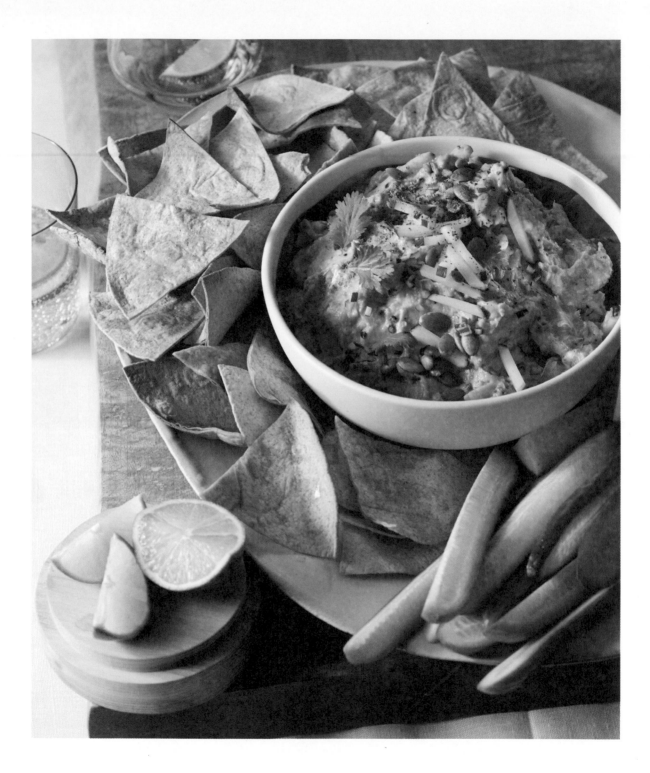

GUACAMOLE

As on the dear old toast (page 38). No need to grill the avocados when you are making the luscious dip full of healthy omega-3 fats. While others enjoy beers topped with lime and salt, I love to enjoy this guac with soda michelada, essentially a salt-rimmed tall glass filled with ice and about 6 tablespoons of fresh lime juice. Served with seltzer water on the side to add as you please, this is a craveable booze-free drink that I have taught many friends when they are in search of a lighter evening. Cucumber slices are my second trick to keep the guac affair a lighter one: along with whole grain baked tortillas, serve the guac with cucumber slices, a perfect crunchy vehicle to the tasty dip.

Makes 3 cups (600 g)

2 avocados

1 teaspoon freshly ground black pepper

1 teaspoon crushed red pepper flakes

1 teaspoon ground cumin

1 teaspoon Himalayan pink salt

3 tablespoons roughly chopped fresh cilantro leaves

2 tablespoons fresh lime juice

1 tablespoon + 1 teaspoon minced red onion

1 ounce (30 g) radish, cut into matchsticks (¼ cup)

2 tablespoons pumpkin seeds, toasted

Lime wedges, optional

Persian cucumber, optional

Whole grain tortilla chips, optional

1. Cut the avocados in half and remove the pit. Holding the halves in your hand, slice the flesh into chunks inside the skin, then scoop out into a bowl, using a spoon.

2. Season with the black pepper, red pepper flakes, cumin, and salt. Mash with the back of a fork, then fold in the cilantro, lime juice, and red onion.

3. Place in a serving bowl and sprinkle with radish and pumpkin seeds.

4. Serve with lime wedges, cucumber slices, or your favorite tortilla chip.

KRAUT

Unlike your traditional kraut made with finely shredded green cabbage, this is roughly shredded purple cabbage, which results in a more rustic sauerkraut with a bright hue that I love to have on hand. My secret flavoring agent is caraway, familiar in flavor to a good seeded rye bread. All you need to do is massage this vegetable and allow it to ferment. Let nature do its thing.

Makes 5 cups (1 kg)

One 2-pound (900 g) head purple cabbage

2 tablespoons Himalayan pink salt

1 teaspoon whole caraway seeds

1 Proviotic

1. Shred the cabbage roughly and place it in a large bowl.

2. Massage the salt and caraway seeds into the cabbage until the cabbage breaks down, 5 to 10 minutes.

3. Place the cabbage in a container or bowl and cover with a clean plate, pressing down. Use a heavy can (try a 32-ounce/905 g can of crushed tomatoes) to weigh down the plate.

4. Place a clean cloth over the top of the container of weighted kraut.

5. Allow the Kraut to ferment at room temperature for 4 to 5 days. It will bubble around the edge of the plate, which means the good bacteria is forming.

6. Strain some of the Kraut liquid, blend it with a Proviotic, and add back to the mixture; this helps keep the Kraut stable in your fridge.

7. Place the Kraut in a large, clean canning jar and store in the fridge for a up to a month.

ROMESCO

This dip, this spread, this moment is everything. I had to make sure it was in the pantry, to add a dollop to a salad, a bowl of grains, or an extra piece of grilled miche bread, next to a bowl of squash soup, as it is that delicious! Despite having an up-and-down relationship with roasted red peppers—stuffed roasted peppers make me queasy, as do slimy grilled vegetables, including peppers, inside panini—I figured out a way to enjoy roasted red peppers. By trial and error, I came to this dip, blitzed with almonds, spices, and bright vinegar. I was sold. The texture is as nourishing as it is satisfying. Being able to enjoy the nutrient-rich red pepper along with protein-packed almonds without its being a chore is essential when living Clean Enough. No matter how good something is for you, if you detest it, it will never be a positive experience.

Makes 2 cups (400 g)

6 ounces (175 g) whole wheat miche sourdough, cut into cubes (1 cup)

2 tablespoons raw almonds

½ large red bell pepper, roasted (see Notes), or ⅔ cup (120 g) store-bought roasted red pepper

½ garlic clove, peeled

2 tablespoons red wine vinegar

2 teaspoons organic tomato paste

½ teaspoon Himalayan pink salt

¼ teaspoon freshly ground black pepper

¼ teaspoon paprika

⅛ teaspoon red pepper flakes

3 tablespoons extra virgin olive oil

1. Preheat the oven to 350°F (180°C) convection.

2. Place the sourdough cubes and almonds on a half sheet pan. Place in the oven to toast for 10 minutes, until golden. Remove from the oven and allow to cool.

3. Place the cooled almonds and sourdough, roasted bell pepper, garlic, vinegar, tomato paste, salt, black pepper, paprika, and red pepper flakes in a high-powered blender. Blend on high speed, scraping down the sides as needed with both a plunger and rubber spatula, until smooth.

4. Add the olive oil and blend to combine, about 10 seconds.

5. Serve immediately.

——————

NOTE

To roast a red pepper, place it on a small sheet pan and set it underneath the broiler in an oven. Allow to blister and char for about 10 minutes on each side. Once completely charred, transfer to a bowl and cover with plastic wrap to steam for a few minutes. Remove the charred skin and discard along with the seeds and green top, reserving the roasted flesh.

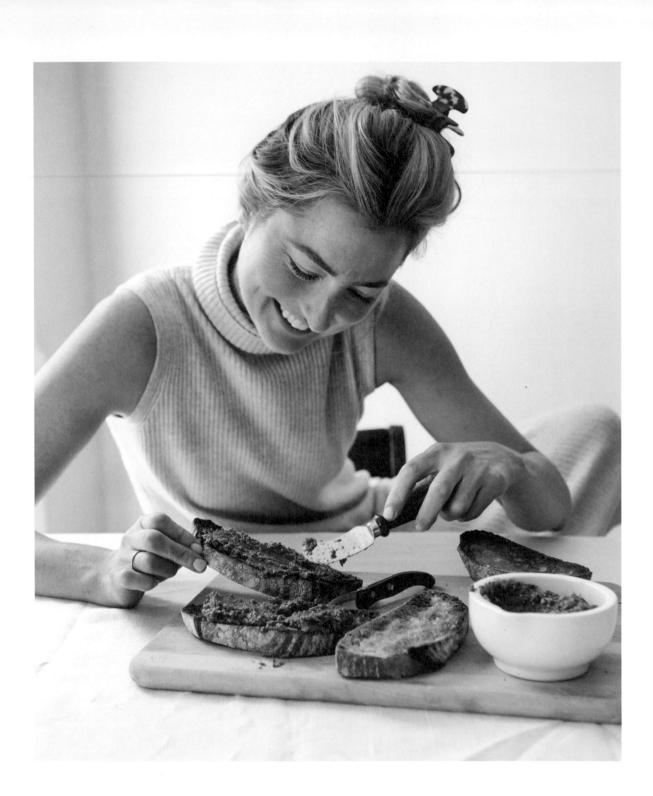

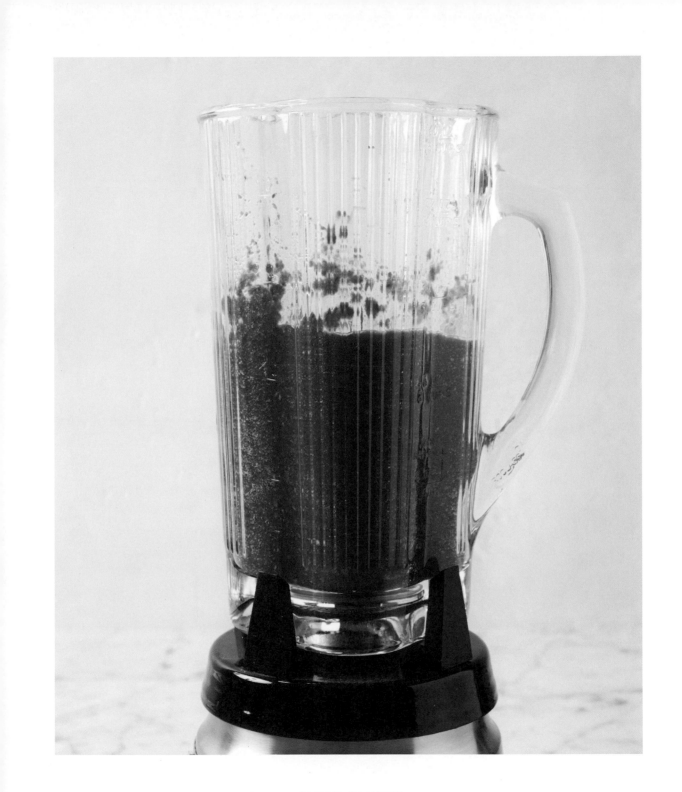

ROOSTER SAUCE

What's pretty fantastic about this sauce is that it is easy to make and has zero fillers and zero added sugar, getting its genius fermenting starter (which is typically table sugar) from prunes, that dried fruit that you never seem to know what to do with. The chiles are what's important here. Red Fresno are about the size of a jalapeño, fairly hot yet full of flavor.

Makes 3 cups (675 g)

5 cups (400 g) red Fresno chiles

3 garlic cloves, peeled

3 or 4 unsulfured prunes, pitted (¾ ounce/20 g)

1 tablespoon Himalayan pink salt

2 tablespoons cider vinegar

1 tablespoon organic tamari (wheat-free soy sauce)

1 Proviotic, cap opened

1. Keeping the green tops intact, snip the stems off the whole chiles, using kitchen scissors.

2. Combine the chiles with the garlic, prunes, and salt in a high-powered blender and blend on high speed until fully pureed.

3. Transfer to a sterilized glass jar (see Notes, page 244). Place the lid on the jar and let sit on the counter at room temperature for 4 days.

4. On the fifth day, stir the mixture with a clean spoon and replace the lid.

5. On the sixth day, stir the mixture with a clean spoon and replace the lid.

6. On the seventh day, transfer the bubbling contents back to a the clean blender, adding the vinegar, tamari, and contents of a Proviotic. Blend on high speed until smooth, about 1½ minutes.

7. Strain the mixture through a fine-mesh strainer, such as a chinois, using a small ladle to push all the paste through, with only the chile seeds remaining.

8. Store in the fridge for up to a month and a half.

ROSE HARISSA

This Tunisian condiment is spicy and elegant, like my highest self. The depth of flavor created lends itself to anything from scrambled or baked eggs to vegetables and grains.

Makes 1 cup (225 g)

1 medium red bell pepper

1 small red onion

2 garlic cloves, peeled

2 red Fresno chiles, seeded (see Rooster Sauce, page 116)

2 tablespoons extra virgin olive oil

¾ teaspoon caraway seeds

¾ teaspoon ground coriander

¾ teaspoon ground cumin

½ teaspoon ground turmeric

1½ tablespoons fresh lemon juice

½ teaspoon freshly ground black pepper

¼ teaspoon Himalayan pink salt

1 tablespoon + 1 teaspoon crushed food-grade rose petals

½ teaspoon rose water (Mymouné preferred)

1. Roast the pepper per the instructions on page 113 for Romesco.

2. Meanwhile, finely chop together the red onion, garlic, and seeded chiles.

3. Heat the olive oil in a skillet over medium-high heat, add the chile mixture, and sauté until dark brown, almost blackened.

4. Meanwhile, in a separate dry skillet, heat the caraway seeds, coriander, cumin, and turmeric over medium heat, until fragrant.

5. Transfer the blackened chile mixture and the spices, roasted bell pepper, lemon juice, salt, and pepper in a high-powered blender and blend until completely smooth.

6. Add the rose petals and rose water and pulse to break down but not puree completely.

7. Store in the fridge for up to two weeks, until ready for use.

PESTO

My happiest moments with pesto involve a glass of red, a cutting board, and a great conversation while I chop away at my pile of herbs, nuts, and spices before dousing it all with olive oil and calling it a day.

The beauty about pesto and this pesto in particular is the freedom to swap out the herbs and nuts. Walnuts work beautifully, but so do toasted hazelnuts. I have been known to add a handful of superspicy baby arugula to my herb mix, or cilantro.

This pesto is for the Mid-August Lunch (page 56) and is also divine dolloped on top of the Coconut Oil Crispy Rice (page 97) and Velvet Beet soup (page 101).

Makes 1 cup (225 g)

1 cup packed (40 g) fresh basil leaves

½ cup packed (50 g) fresh mint leaves

½ cup packed (30 g) fresh parsley leaves

1 garlic clove

¼ cup (25 g) pine nuts (toasted or raw, depending on your preference)

½ teaspoon grated lemon zest

1 teaspoon Himalayan pink salt

½ teaspoon freshly ground black pepper

⅓ cup (80 ml) extra virgin olive oil

1 tablespoon fresh lemon juice

1. Pile all the herbs on your cutting board along with the garlic and chop roughly.

2. At this point you can transfer to a mortar and pestle along with the nuts, lemon zest, salt, and pepper, and begin to mash with the oil, seasoning with the lemon juice at the end.

3. Alternatively, you can transfer the mixture to a food processor to pulse with the lemon juice and stream in the oil, or you can make a finer puree by using a high-speed blender, streaming in the olive oil.

4. Finally, you can go ditch all these tools and finish by hand. Continue chopping the herbs with the garlic, nuts, and lemon zest until very fine and then stir in the salt and pepper. Transfer to a bowl and stir in the lemon juice and olive oil there, as to not make a further mess of your cutting board.

II

—

ENOUGH

Welcome to the Sweeter Side

Being afraid of your own creative talent is something I know all too well. After years of swinging between hiding from a slice of cake, rewarding my suppressed emotions with gelato, denying myself a treat when it was wholly acceptable, battling myself when my rear end expanded and equally when it flattened, I had to say to myself, *Enough is enough.* I had to accept my perfectionist tendencies and embrace my pursuit of health and the joy that clean nutrition habits bring me, while understanding that my life at its flexible and optimum state included balance and acceptance, not just broccoli. Realizing that I am no longer a veggie-obsessed outsider among my sweet peers has provided even more motivation to continue honing my take on the sweet craft while maintaining a sound body and mind.

I know that my passion in life is desserts, so I've made it my mission to live whole and Clean *Enough* to enjoy them without letting them take over my health. In practice having found this personal freedom with food and taking responsibility for what I put in my body has made my favorite molasses cookie moments possible. Because I don't approach these moments with guilt, they do negatively impact my health; rather, they're balanced by healthy daily habits. Even if I fall out of alignment, I know that I have the ability to move with it, ask why and remind myself that it's all about consistency and, frankly, never really about that chocolate chip cookie.

This is what living Clean Enough means to me: the clean and dirty sides of your personal wellness strategy. I can enjoy desserts just "enough" because my lifestyle honors treats for what they are: Memorable moments that happen sometimes, in great company, and, in my world, are often of the sweeter persuasion. Understanding that real, whole foods fuel my body and brain with vitamins and minerals; foods that fight off disease, infections, depression, hormone imbalances, digestive issues, and more; that serve as preventative medicine we all need to live to our potential. I enjoy them well enough on their own, but I can't claim perfection in seeking only these foods every moment of my life.

The ultimate Clean requires having peace around all types of food.

At this point, with the arsenal of savory, nutrient-rich whole meals just behind you in this food journey, I hope that you feel confident to take on the sweeter side, too. Take your time, make what elicits a grin (and please make enough to share). You do not need dessert: You have dessert because it is special and when made with loving hands, it always seems to taste that much better. I guarantee that you will build some differentiating skills as you explore these recipes and techniques with patience. All are achievable, and with practice you will strengthen your artistic and technical muscles. Creating your Enough with an exacting hand lies ahead.

I believe there is a perfect dessert for every moment, and offered here are what I hope are best of class: the cookies, pies, tarts, messes, meringues, puddings, sauces, and the like that I have organically developed over time—from straightforward classics, to variations with a few nuances, to the quirky creations that have come from accidental moments (e.g., my twin loves of watching Wimbledon while contemplating pie). One of the greatest things about desserts is the mindfulness required to make each component. Yes, you are making a treat and you are making it deliberately strengthening skills that will lead to future creative freedom. Show up to your next dinner party with a pile of one of these cookies and a tub of ice cream and sit at the counter with your friends, making them ice cream sammies. Make a batch of the scones for your next brunch, split in half and swathed with clotted cream and preserves, native style. You will remember what the good life tastes like. Love and being mindful are running themes here. Embrace them; along with butter, flour, sugar, and eggs, and always lick the bowl clean.

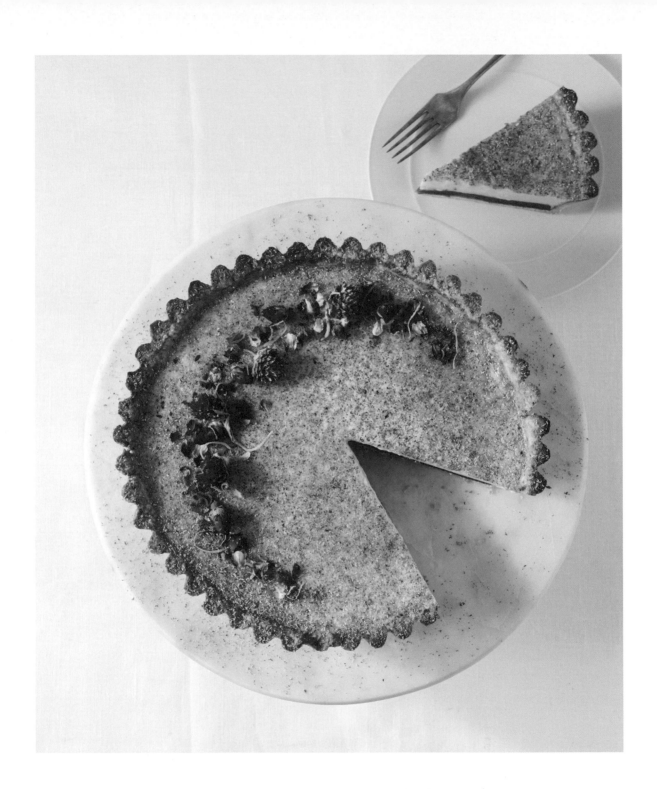

SWEET BEGINNINGS

It all started when I failed to make the Starlight White Cake from the orange *Betty Crocker Cookbook* every week of my tenth year. *Who is Betty Crocker, anyway?* I thought each time she bested me at that simplest of recipes. *What does she have that I don't?* I now know she's a figment of a publisher's imagination. My lack of focus and patience was represented in all of the failed white cakes that crumbled out of the steamy pans attempting to cool briefly outside in the New England winter. I would go with the still-warm cake only to unmold it into a pile of, you guessed it, still-warm cake crumbs. Needless to say, these Starlight White Cakes remained beyond disappointing and reflected my expectation of perfection from myself; patience was something I thought was a virtue I was missing, rather than a learned skill.

Then came a day when the cooled cake sprung from the pan intact: a disk of pale white glory. I had mastered the Starlight White Cake! Achieving this cake gave me such satisfaction that I became hooked on the process. I began to bake fiendishly and fed people my creations with the right balance of determination and quirkiness that would push me upward into the executive ranks of New York City. Day after day I got by on the thrill of removing a pan from the oven, plating it just so, and serving it with great fervor to my customers: Watching them enjoy what I hoped would be a moment of pure joy was the equivalent of a thousand sugar rushes, and then some.

From Betty Crocker to Camp Bement, the sleepaway summer camp representing the formative years of youth, the engine for dessert-making had started. As young teens in the Adventure Base program, we would be responsible for retrieving and cooking all our own food—sometimes over a fire, sometimes on the side of a mountain during a multiday traverse. Adventure Base taught me a lot about the balance of independence and working together as a team, an awareness that is essential as you move through your adult life and write a cookbook, for example. Adventure Base also had me wandering into the camp's kitchen, getting to know the staff and the lay of the land. This ultimately led me to working in the kitchen during the weekends in the off-season. The Bement kitchen was the initiation, leading me to craft hundreds of loaves of Pullman bread, cookies, and desserts for both campers and off-season conference groups. I pored over books such as the original *Gotham Bar and Grill Cookbook*, *The Secrets of Baking*, and *Culinary Artistry*, all foreshadowing my future. I became obsessed with temperatures and textures, from warm white chocolate paired with cool strawberries to silky fudge slipped over crispy *pâte à choux* with cool and creamy ice cream. All of this baking fueled me to attend culinary school and thus begin my road to pastry chef-dom.

Close to graduation was a test in perseverance, calling Spago's bakeshop hoping to speak to chef Sherry Yard and being told to call back in an hour, in fifteen minutes, Chef Sherry is frosting a cake, call back tomorrow. I thought I was being tested.

I finally got hold of the pink chef coat–wearing dynamo. "When can you start?" she said. I was floored, sitting in a parking lot somewhere, with a timer at the ready in case she asked me to call back in five. I flew to the West Coast the day after I graduated from FCI and jumped right in, all the while still being south of a legal drinking age. I was in need of a mentor and Sherry not only taught me about pluots and Persian mulberries, she taught me how to assemble a cookbook; run charity events; pack and ship anything, from gallons of ice cream to delicate blown sugar, anywhere; how to respect your products; appreciate good relationships; about the mystical wonders of kombucha; how to fall in love at any age; and how to measure your curtains so they fall before a window like a lady's dress.

London brought me to the famed Berkeley Hotel, where Marcus Wareing and Gordon Ramsay slayed perfectly executed British desserts. SBE Restaurants brought me into the realm of pastry artistry with the Wolfgang Puck empire never falling out of orbit.

Landing back in New York as the founding pastry chef of the Breslin at the Ace Hotel, I worked tirelessly to harmonize meringues with liqueurs, and lace dangerous liquid velvet drinks with spiced sprits. I was at the epicenter of a revolution in the NoMad (north of Madison Square Park) area of New York, where the word *disruptive* was being used to describe chef-driven ingredient-focused concepts and a certain new understated cool in what people were seeking with food, drink, art, and culture. Hyatt hotels exposed me to corporate structure, scale, and creative freedom. The Hyatt also supported me through my *Top Chef* endeavors and desire to push my mind to think strategically and creatively outside of a kitchen. I was on reality TV, doing consulting, running the Pastry Program, on the Design Thinking Team, volunteering and helping friends open a restaurant in Kentucky on the weekends. I am exhausted even writing about it!

Top Chef: Just Desserts was a fairly remarkable period of time. I had no intention of being a reality maven; that had been a bucket-list item, as my voice and perspective were not yet fully baked enough to pursue any sort of spotlight. Besides lifelong friendships, personal encouragement to fight for what I believe in, and an ultimate test of grace under pressure, my biggest takeaway was the power of removing distractions giving way for creative freedom and execution. I daresay I would have never thought to create an edible dripping beehive or interactive carrot cake garden if I had the influence of work, life, New York, my cell phone, and the like happening in parallel. When you are left to dig deep, exciting things can happen.

And then, there was Max Brenner. A long whirlwind of global travel, chocolate milkshakes, and matcha lattes before they were a thing. Max Brenner made me far more culturally aware and curious. I gained many skills, and primarily what I got and was after was understanding how to live as a citizen of the world, respecting and interacting with everyone from a Russian dishwasher to a Japanese CEO.

Along this journey. my taste in sweets has been evolving but has maintained its combination of elegance and casual flair. The incredible people and experiences on the sweet side of my life have continued to support my health-focused endeavors. The synchronicity I have encountered is not by accident and, rather, shows the interconnectedness experienced when you are on the right path. Being purpose-driven has brought me closer to that delicious combination of wants and needs, and the beautiful influencers have supported every blended coconut smoothie and roasted fish with the same vigor that they supported baked Alaska on a stick and other moments of pure imagination.

IN THE ICEBOX

Baking can be incredibly intimidating for some, even master cooks I've worked and studied with. If that's you, or even if it's not, it's a good thing you have this book! Baking Clean Enough means simplifying and demystifying what you thought you couldn't do.

For *all* my ingredients, including the basics, namely flour, butter, sugar and eggs, I purchase the highest quality I can afford, relying heavily on organic and unbleached products. The unrefined ingredients do slightly affect the texture, rendering slightly heartier results than those using ultrarefined ingredients. This is not an approach to making desserts healthy: Treats are not viewed as nutritionally balanced, but rather as emotional nutrition, so the higher quality, the better. This also means I'm creating the best version of a dessert I can achieve, sharing moments that are just Enough.

Build your pantry slowly over time by selecting a new recipe and reading it start to finish before you even write a shopping list or go to the store to acquire the ingredients that often can be used again for another recipe in the book.

You will find that some ingredients, such as cinnamon, honey, and rose water, are used in both savory and sweet applications. If there is a question regarding a sweet ingredient, be sure to also reference the savory glossary on page 2. Support your local businesses first by purchasing spices and floral waters from spice stores (I proudly support Kalustyan's in New York City). All of these ingredients can be purchased at Whole Foods with the exception of a few that can be filled in by Amazon, such as my favorite variety of rose water. Do not feel beholden to any brands that I mention; rather, make the best choices for you at the grocery store!

Baking Powder: Sodium bicarbonate or baking soda with the acid added needed to activate the chemical leavening properties of the soda. Cream of tartar is often the acid that is used in this blend. Classified as a chemical leavener, gives rise to pastries when combined activated with moisture and heat. This ingredient is what gives extra rise to the whipped Pan di Spagna batter.

Baking Soda: Sodium bicarbonate, classified as a chemical leavener, gives rise to pastries when combined with acidic ingredients in the recipe. For example, brown sugar, used in the Generous Chocolate Chunk Cookies, is more acidic than granulated cane sugar, and often the right balance for baking soda without the need for baking powder, which already has an acid added to the product.

Bread Starter: Made simply from flour and water and with an added aroma agent, such as fragrant grapes or figs (optional). This mixture is allowed to sit and ferment at room temperature over the course of two weeks, fed with fresh water and flour intermittently, until live bacteria, developing lactic acid, create a natural leavening ability. Bread starter will last as long as it is fed, replenishing the food source of water and flour for continued live cultures. The starter is an essential component to most of the breads in *Clean Enough*, adding flavor and leavening to the dough.

Butter: Choose organic unsalted butter for these sweet recipes. Alternatives are grass-fed butter, with a more intense flavor, and European butter, with a higher fat content that makes the flavor so intense it almost tastes fake. Goat's milk butter is from a completely different animal, and more opaque in color and fattier or greasier in texture.

Candied Fennel Seeds: A traditional confection in Indian cuisine, where humble fennel seeds are thinly coated in colored sugar. I use candied fennel seeds in place of rainbow sprinkles in my It's My Birthday Milkshake as well as for decorations on cakes and other sweets. They can easily be purchased at an Indian market or online.

Chocolate: I love Michel Cluizel and Guittard brands; both are accessible for the home cook either at Whole Foods or from Amazon. Do not feel that you can't make the recipes without these! Explore the chocolate that is available to you. From chocolate bar frosting, to cookies, tarts, milkshakes, and sauces, chocolate brings a distinct and strong flavor as well as texture to desserts.

Chocolate is a beautiful mass made from the fruit pod of the cacao tree. Chocolate involves a multistep process to go from pod to bar, resulting in a variety of milk

and dark chocolate varieties along with cocoa powder. The fat from the cacao is also utilized to make deliciously sweet white chocolate.

Milk chocolate runs approximately 31 percent cocoa solids with the inclusion of sugar, cocoa butter, and milk powder.

Bittersweet dark chocolate runs approximately 60 to 64 percent cocoa solids with *dark chocolate* in the 70 to 72 percent cocoa solids ballpark. I find that the higher the cocoa solids, the greater the potential for the chocolate to be chalkier when used for baking or eating. The lower the percentage of cocoa solids, the higher percentage of sugar, thus a sweeter and less bitter chocolate.

One hundred percent chocolate would denote 100 percent cocoa solids without any added sugar. This variety of chocolate is intense and is to be used as an ingredient within a recipe.

White chocolate is not chocolate at all! Rather, it is a mixture of milk solids, vanilla, sugar, and cocoa butter. Delicious and added as a creamy sweetener in the Coconut Cake.

Cocoa powder are cocoa solids without added fat or sugar. *Extra brut* denotes a deep, dark cocoa powder, whereas alkalized, or Dutch, processes result in a lighter cocoa. While I prefer extra brut, do not be afraid to use what you have.

When chocolate as an ingredient is listed as a wafer, this refers to melting chocolate couverture disks (rather than bar chocolate or chips), aka buttons or pastilles/pistoles.

Cinnamon: Ceylon cinnamon is considered "true" cinnamon: pure and spicy, carrying that hot and sweet flavor through any recipe. Cassia, while having a cinnamon aroma, is more bitter and often has additives. Ceylon cinnamon is what makes Jim Welu's Cinnamon Ice Cream as well as the molasses cookies spicy warm and sweet.

Condensed Milk (Sweetened): Milk that has been reduced to a thick syrup and sweetened. It offers creaminess, sweetness, and moisture to recipes. When it is further cooked to the point of browning the milk solids, you get a sauce called dulce de leche—essentially caramelized condensed milk.

Flour

- **All-Purpose:** A standard wheat flour that I purchase organic and unbleached. All-purpose flour is the go-to for most recipes, offering structure and strength without the delicacy of pastry flour or strength of bread flour.

- **Bread:** Organic wheat flour with a high amount of gluten, bread flour gives strength to doughs for heartier breakfast pastries and breads. Gluten, the protein found in wheat flour, develops when mixed with water and kneaded in the bread-making process. A strong dough brings structure for yeast to eat the dough's sugars and release gas, thus making the bread rise.

- **Pastry:** Also known as cake flour, pastry flour is fine wheat flour that has the lowest amount of gluten (wheat protein) of all of the flours used in this book. This creates a more tender crumb in recipes such as the shortbread cookies.

Fruits and Vegetables

- **Freeze-Dried Fruit/Berries:** Freeze-drying is a process by which all water is extracted from a product while maintaining a majority of the structure of an ingredient, unlike processed dried fruit, which shrinks the original fresh product.

- **Quince:** A beautiful fruit that looks slightly similar to a green apple. When raw, the texture is spongy and the taste sour. When peeled and poached, quince turns a bright pink with a soft unctuous texture and a sweet flavor and aroma. Perfect as a tart filling or cooked further to be made into a paste often served on a cheese board.

- **Raisins:** There is a multitude of varieties of golden or yellow raisins, each with its own level of sweetness and tartness. Dark raisins, Thompson, red flame, and currants also range in size, depth of rich brown sugar flavor, and tartness. Have fun with raisins and buy organic, which do not contain the preservative sulfur dioxide.

Halva: Halva is a beautiful confection made of sugar and tahini paste, often jazzed up with honey or additional nuts. Halva is sold in block form and is a melt-in-your-mouth (thanks to the high fat content of sesame seeds) yet crumbly treat. You would purchase it as you would American fudge—wrapped in wax paper—but it is rich like British brown sugar and butter fudge. Halva also comes in a thread variety, where it looks almost like loose cotton or fabric. If you can find this, buy it and eat it right away!

Heavy Cream: Finding true heavy cream can be confusing among the rows of its cousins, light cream and whipping cream, in American dairy sections. Light cream has had some of the fat removed, and is of no use to me in baking. Whipping cream has had stabilizers added, which prevent the cream from losing volume if it sits after whipping. I also avoid this and opt for great local organic heavy cream that tastes rich and thick even without added vanilla, sugar, or other flavors. A staple whipped cream, whipped anywhere from soft to stiff peaks, is called for throughout the book as both a topping and an ingredient.

Honey: Honey is one of my favorite things in life, and is used in Clean applications such as the Luxury Granola, along with such Enough recipes as the coveted Honey Butter. High-quality honey is just that: raw, and full of the rich floral notes, such as orange blossom, clover, and lavender, that processing can eliminate. The flavor depends on where it has been cultivated, in a way that could be related to wines and grapes taking on the characteristics of the terrain. My go-to honey is always orange blossom—pale, floral, and sweet.

Lyle's Golden Syrup: Hailing from the UK, this is an invert sugar syrup made during the sugar refining process. It has a light amber color and rich flavor and a viscosity similar to that of honey.

Maple Syrup: Sap that has been tapped from maple trees and boiled down, evaporating the water and concentrating the sugars to form an amber syrup. Rich with maple flavor and full of minerals, this is a natural liquid sugar that is not as viscous as honey but very sweet and uniquely flavorful. Maple syrup acts as a topping to sweet breakfast dishes as well as an ingredient in simple syrups, poaching liquids, and warm beverages in this book.

Mascarpone: Italian cream cheese, with a sweeter flavor than its American counterpart and made without additives or thickeners.

Milk Powder: Milk powder is not trying to fool anyone with its name. It's added to ice cream bases to provide protein and richness without the need for more (or any) cream and egg yolks. Make sure that you purchase a high-quality organic milk powder, as you would a high-quality organic milk with a cream line.

Molasses: Blackstrap molasses is the richest, darkest version of molasses, the final concentrated by-product when sugar is completely extracted from sugarcane to crystallize into what we know as granulated sugar. Molasses is spicy and intense, full of minerals, and adds depth of flavor and moisture to recipes.

Orange Blossom Water: Has the aroma and flavor of a very floral, zested orange. Perfectly complements recipes calling for orange zest or juice and otherwise adds a pleasant bright floral note to all sweets. I love the Mymouné variety, which adds a beautiful flavor to the date puree used in the Silk Road Custard Tart.

Pectin: Extracted from the seeds of apples, pectin, when heated, thickens the liquid released from fruit in the process of making preserves, jams, and jellies. This helps create a spreadable consistency when placed on toasts or streaked into creams. Pectin can clump easily. I recommend combining the measured amount with sugar to disperse the particles before shaking it into the liquid while whisking.

Pimm's: A citrusy, spicy gin-based liqueur traditionally used for a "Pimm's cup," a summer cocktail with either lemonade or ginger ale and refreshing garnishes such as cucumbers, strawberries, and mint.

Pistachios: Many varieties are available. California pistachios are a bright and hearty green and are what you will traditionally see used in recipes that call for whole nuts. Persian pistachios have a purple and green hue; they are absolutely beautiful with a softer flavor. Sicilian pistachios are bright green, creamy, and nutty (and slightly coconutty to me). I purchase my Sicilian pistachios whole and shelled (and not in paste form), as not all pistachio pastes are created equal. If you do not live in a town or a city with a great spice, Indian, Middle Eastern, or Italian market, you can purchase Sicilians online. Mind you, these are the most expensive of the pistachio bunch! Treat them as you would saffron—use just enough.

Praline Paste: A paste made from deeply roasted hazelnuts and dark amber caramelized sugar ground together. Praline paste imparts a rich hazelnut flavor and is often used as an ingredient in ice creams, cakes, and candies. The intensity of praline paste is far deeper than a nut butter like almond or peanut butter. That is, you can make hazelnut butter from plain hazelnuts, but it's unlike the unique flavor of praline. Praline paste can be store-bought, but as I mention in the Praline Paste recipe, it is best to make your own.

Ricotta: A soft curd cheese that comes in varying depths of flavor as well as fat contents, depending on the milk used. Low-fat basic ricotta generally falls flat on flavor. For the sweet recipes, be sure to purchase whole-milk ricotta, preferably sheep's milk; local will often yield better results, too, as the curds are creamier with more flavor.

Sugar

- **Confectioners':** Also known as 10X, icing sugar, or powdered sugar, confectioners' sugar is finely ground sugar with a small portion of cornstarch added to prevent clumping. Always make sure to sift it even if the recipe does not call for this step.

- **Granulated Cane:** The organic variety used in this book is less refined than white granulated table sugar and made exclusively from sugarcane. The granules are slightly larger, with a touch of the molasses tones of the natural sugar intact. Organic granulated cane sugar weighs more, cup for cup, than refined white granulated sugar. The dessert recipes in *Clean Enough* call for the organic variety, so use organic cane sugar and follow the weight measurements for best results.

- **Light Brown:** Granulated cane sugar that is moistened with molasses, offering a complex and rich base to pastries. Dark brown sugar is also available, which simply denotes a greater amount of molasses being added. In many countries, brown sugar is not available; rather, a portion of high-quality molasses should be added to a tub of granulated sugar in a food processor to create a batch of brown sugar.

Vanilla: Vanilla is a go-to familiar flavor that rounds out the flavor and weight of fat and sugar. In this book, it comes in the form of extract, whole bean, scraped seeds, or bean paste. Madagascar vanilla is the most common, and the one I always use to bake. I have had affairs with Tahitian vanilla, though, which is more floral and certainly more expensive and difficult to acquire.

Yeast (Instant): Classified as an organic leavener, instant yeast is the fastest-acting, texturally fine yeast available to the general public. Fresh yeast cakes require refrigeration; dried active yeast needs time to "bloom," or awaken the dormant culture; and instant yeast simply needs moisture to activate. Salt can easily kill yeast, with its harsh pH, which is why salt is often not immediately added to recipes until after the initial blooming and feeding. Salt, however, is essential to the texture and flavor of dough and balances out yeast growth and feeding.

TOOLS OF THE TRADE

I like to keep my tool kit simple in the world of sweets, allowing me to bake anywhere and everywhere. Cabin in the woods? Fully decked-out pro kitchen with an expansive island? An NYC-apartment-size mini oven with no counter space? I accept any and all challenges. I have had to sift flour using a pasta colander in my formative days and am just as comfortable with that as I am with a hand-cranked sifting device. Feel confident using what you have along with me.

That being said, I have two tasks that I implore you to complete before making another move, ensuring success with *Clean Enough*.

Read. The. Recipe.

My first piece of advice will change your approach to baking forever: Before you do anything—buy anything, turn the oven on, get out a mixer, invite your friends over—read the recipe from top to bottom. Read the headnote, yield, baking temperature, ingredient list, all the directions in their entirety, serving suggestions, and notes, then read them again. Let the story of what you're about to bake unfold as sweetly as the flavors do upon first bite. All of a sudden, that daunting layer cake just became logical and possible.

Acquire. A. Digital. Scale.

My second piece of advice is to buy a digital scale. There is nothing easier and more exact than a scale. Baking is a science, whereas cooking, while still a science (remember all those nutrition facts from part 1? That's science), is a far more casual affair. Scales come in all shapes, sizes, and price points, so you really have no excuse if you want to have your cake and eat it, too.

Now, less urgent, but still transformative, tools . . .

Balloon Whisk: The base of this whisk is larger and more bulbous than a typical hand whisk, allowing you to incorporate more air into hand-whipped meringue or cream and also to delicately fold flour into cake batters with ease and efficiency. While you can rely on your stand mixer's whisk attachment, I think that having a balloon whisk on hand always helps for the final fold, ensuring no flour clumps are left and batters are not deflated, as well as allowing you to whip smaller portions of creams without turning on a machine.

Bench Scraper: A blunt metal handheld scraper is multipurpose, including for cutting portions of dough for buns, scraping ingredients off your work surface into a bowl, and cleaning up your work surface after you have rolled bread, measured multiple recipes, and have smatterings of sticky mess. (It can serve the same purpose in all varieties of veggie prep.) The blunt side can also function to smooth the sides of a frosted cake while spinning it on a cake stand.

Bowl Scraper: A small, plastic handheld scraper that generally comes in a standard rounded 4 x 6-inch (10 x 15 cm) rectangle that is perfect for removing the last bits of batter from a mixing bowl, folding cake batter, or scooping out a small portion of frosting or curd for a filling. This is a multiuse tool that I hoard and swear by.

Convection Oven: A convection oven circulates air, baking and cooking recipes more quickly, evenly, and at a lower heat than a standard still oven. If you are using a still oven, increase the baking temperatures by 25 degrees Fahrenheit (20 degrees Celsius) and increase baking times by about 15 minutes.

Digital Thermometer: A digital thermometer that can go to 400°F (200°C) is a great addition to your toolbox. This helps determine the accurate cooking of egg-based custards, without allowing them to scramble, as well as making sure that hot sugar syrup is combined at the right moment with whipping egg white for Italian Meringue. Your thermometer does not need to be expensive. It is important to never submerge the entire tool in liquid, just the temperature measuring stick.

Fine-Mesh Strainer: A fine-mesh strainer called a chinois is cone shaped and can strain anything from a lemon curd or soup to fruit puree and nut milk. The secret to using a fine-mesh chinois is to use a small ladle that fits snugly in the tip of the cone, to press out all the liquid and leave only the

solid remains. A chinois can be a pricey purchase, as this is a high-quality tool, so an alternative is an almond milk bag or cheesecloth draped in a basket sifter.

A Good Spoon: A great tool, not just a vehicle for eating. Look for one larger and less round than a soupspoon yet smaller than a serving spoon. I encourage you to find your spoon. The best schmears, swooshes, drizzles, and dollops will come from your spoon, creating treats that cry out "devour me!" for these casual techniques create effortlessly delicious desserts.

High-Powered Blender: Highly utilized in both the Clean and Enough sections of the book, a high-speed blender will be your go-to for all smoothies, sauces, soups, and many new mixtures to come. You can use a standard blender or another variety of high-speed blender, but I do love and recommend Vitamix. There is a low setting with an adjustable speed as well as the high setting that will create the smoothest purees and tightest emulsifications of sauces imaginable. I keep my Vitamix on my counter now as I use it habitually for my collagen-reinforced morning beverages as well as for quick dinners when I return home from work.

Ice Cream Machine: At-home ice-cream machines come in a variety of styles and prices. There are vessels that you can freeze before adding your ice cream base and then cranking by hand. There are also electric varieties that allow you to freeze an insulated chamber and then place it back on the machine with the ice cream base and it will paddle the liquid until it freezes. More expensive at-home varieties have their own compressor that freezes the chamber as the ice cream base is paddled. I have the best luck with an electric ice cream machine that requires me to freeze the insulated chamber prior to "spinning" or churning the ice cream base to frozen. When I have room in my freezer, I tend to just keep the ice cream barrel in there as it takes overnight to freeze.

Immersion Blender: Also called a stick blender, this is a handheld wand with a blender at one end that is a great tool for emulsifying ganaches or sauces and creating purees without transferring a mixture to a standard or high-powered blender. It also allows you to control any air incorporation because when the blender head is completely submerged into a liquid, no additional air gets incorporated. The result is a dense and silky ganache, with a smooth, even elastic texture. Also extremely useful for soups and dips.

Large, Heatproof Spatula: This is a plastic-handled, rubber-based flexible spatula that will not melt when placed on a hot pan. Large rubber spatulas are perfect for anything from folding cake batters to scraping the bottom of a mixing bowl or saucepot, as well as scraping the remains of batters and frosting from vessels.

Mini Blowtorch: There is nothing quite like torched meringue or a crispy sugared top on a crème brûlée. I suggest grabbing a mini blowtorch from a kitchen store. A larger blowtorch from a home improvement store will also work but can be extremely dangerous! In a pinch, a broiler can be used to torch meringue as well as blacken your toasted Italian cheesecake.

Offset Spatula: Ideally with a wooden handle and metal scraper, this will save you when spreading cake batter or frosting your chocolate cake. The offset angle allows you to stay in control of the tool without dragging the side of your hand through whatever you are spreading. Mini offsets are great tools for spreading fillings inside of the Biancas (page 145) and smoothing the final touches of your Pan di Spagna (page 156) after you have used a larger offset to do the initial spread.

Quarter and Half Sheet Pans: Standard half sheet pans (13 x 18 inch/33 x 45.5 cm) are made of aluminum and fit into most standard home ovens. Quarter sheet pans (9 x 13 inch/23 x 33 cm) are half the size of standard half sheet pans. Both are rectangular with 1-inch (2.5 cm) sides, perfect for baking cookies or sheet cakes.

Scale: Again, please, buy a digital scale! They come in all shapes, sizes, colors, and price points. Buy a scale that measures in grams as well as ounces and can count individual grams rather than increments of 10 grams. You will find your sweet world changed when you start measuring all of your ingredients on a scale. You will have more accurate outcomes, more ease preparing to bake, and fewer containers used to measure each component.

Serrated Knife: Saves a lot of grief when cutting cooled cakes in half for layering/frosting purposes. The teeth of the serrated knife allow you to break through the crumb structure of breads and cakes by dispersing pressure while cutting. A blunt knife can be used but can sometimes push together the crumb structure rather than cut through it. You can compare it to the difference between sawing a tree and taking an ax to it.

Silicone Mat: A nonstick reusable mat that can be used to line sheet pans for baking. These are great investments as they are reusable and help ensure even spreading of cookies.

Springform Pan: A baking pan with a hinged side allowing expansion of the rim, thus releasing the sides and giving access to the removable bottom. I recommend getting a pan that is 11 inches (28 cm) in diameter for these recipes, which allows for accurate and even baking of low-height cakes. Springform pans are often used for cheesecakes, given their moist batter, but I use them for flour-based cakes as well.

Stand Mixer: A countertop mixer with a removable bowl and hinged head allowing for easy scraping, mixing, and whipping. Stand mixers come with a standard set of attachments, including a paddle for creaming such items as butter and sugar for cookie dough, a whisk for whipping eggs or cream, and a hook for kneading bread dough. Some models additionally have another space on the front of the machine for additional attachments, such as an oat mill for fresh oats, a pasta roller, or even a grinder. While it is an investment, if you plan on baking, I highly suggest having a KitchenAid brand stand mixer in your home.

Tart Pan: A fluted pan made of heavy aluminum with a removable bottom, making it easier to pop the completed tart out without breaking the delicate crust. These come in a variety of diameters, but I recommend a pan that is 9 inches (23 cm) in diameter and more than 2 inches (5 cm deep) or 10 or 11 inches (25.5 or 28 cm) in diameter and 1½ inches (4 cm) deep for these recipes. They are generally made of heavy aluminum with the removable bottom.

BASIC TECHNIQUES

The desserts here are all achievable by any person, regardless of the starting skill set. Eventually, though, you will want to master these key baking techniques that will up your creative potential and allow ease moving through a variety of recipes. Please refer back to this section if you need an *aha* moment, and always read the recipes from start to finish before you do a thing. This will make you feel more comfortable with your journey, and the destination that much sweeter. *Enjoy the journey!*

Blanchir: Whipping whole eggs or egg yolks with sugar, dissolving the sugar into the eggs and thickening the egg yolk mixture to denature the protein and fat structure of the egg. This results in a creamy and thick pale yellow mixture of egg and sugar paste that allow the eggs' incredible bonding properties to incorporate into custards and other mixtures. After cooking, the result is an even and softly set mixture with a smooth mouthfeel.

Blind Baking: Baking a crust that will eventually hold a filling with a false filling. This allows the crust to bake either partially or fully, leaving space for the filling before baking again or chilling.

Creaming: Paddling butter and sugar together, which creates an emulsified, homogenous consistency. The fat breaks down the sugar granules and coats them, creating an even dispersion of sugar and fat, textural essentials. When you overcream your butter, cookies will often fall flat, whereas undercreamed butter results in rounder cookies that do not spread as much and have a harder texture.

Dry Caramel: Sugar cooked until it goes through all of the stages of hardening—soft ball, soft crack, hard ball, and hard crack—before the chemical structure of the sugar reverses, browning the sucrose to create a nutty flavor known as caramel. When you take granulated sugar and heat it without the incorporation of additional ingredients, such as water, the sugar melts easily on its own. Dry caramel is made by gradually melting granulated cane sugar in a pan or pot that is dry and free of debris that can cause the fragile melted sugar to seize and crystallize. Eventually the liquid sugar will bubble slightly and begin to brown, first to a light amber that is still sweet, then a medium amber that is less sweet and nuttier, and finally to a dark amber that is slightly bitter.

Emulsifying: Evenly blending two opposing mixtures together, creating a tight elastic core or emulsification. For example, solid chocolate and a liquid, such as heavy cream, do not incorporate easily on their own. When combined at a warm, melted state and stirred continuously from the center, forming the beginning of the bond, the two mixtures will come together evenly and homogenously to form a smooth mixture that has the qualities of both heavy cream and melted chocolate, but now combined.

Folding: Mixing gently while maintaining volume. Using a large spatula or balloon whisk, you cut down the center of a bowl, then turn the spatula or whisk over as you drag through the mixture back out toward the sides. You continue to fold the bottom of the batter up to the top while turning the bowl continuously. This cut-and-fold motion, while turning, allows for even, delicate mixing.

Lamination: Mechanical leavening, placing layers of butter in between layers of dough. In a hot oven, the butter will melt and the small amount of water in the butter will create steam that will give rise to the dough product in the oven. Shaggy dough creates a rough lamination on its own because of the layering process. You can achieve even lamination by making a strong and evenly mixed dough and placing whole butter pats directly on top of the dough. When the dough is folded either in half or over and over, this creates thin layers of butter between the dough. This mixture is strong enough to hold its structure when steam is released, causing the dough to pouf up and hold as the butter layers melt. Think of buttering a piece of bread: If you folded the bread into a trifold you would end up with multiple layers of bread and butter versus one layer of bread and one layer of butter.

Nappage: Cooking a custard just until the proteins in eggs or egg yolks sets the liquid, so the mixture is able to coat the back of a spoon without dripping. This is achieved at 180°F (82°C). When you overheat a gentle custard set by eggs, the proteins further tighten and the liquid or water surrounding the proteins cannot be held or stabilized by the eggs. This results in a clumpy mixture of tight egg protein with liquid floating around it rather than with it.

Sifting: Flour can often have clumps that will not break down on their own in batters as well as highly concentrated baking powder and baking soda do. Sifting dry ingredients in a mesh basket allows these mixtures, of varying strength and effect on the finished baked product, to mix together; it removes clumps, and aerates, making the incorporation into the wet mixture far easier.

Tempering: The act of introducing a hot substance to a cooler, sensitive substance in small amounts to bring the sensitive substance up in temperature, thus meeting the hot substance

halfway. When you introduce a small amount of hot liquid to eggs that can easily scramble, for instance, you lessen the chances of scrambling all the eggs when adding the slightly warmed eggs to the final hot liquid.

Whipping: Incorporating air into a liquid or mixture that can hold volume; eggs, heavy cream, and egg whites are great examples. By whipping at a medium intensity, you build a stable bubble network, increasing the volume of the original dense substance. When you whip on high speed immediately, the bubbles are larger and inherently more fragile. The smaller and more even the air bubbles that are incorporated, the more stable the whipped product is. When a mixture is whipped on medium and then high speed to achieve maximum volume, it is a wise idea to then return the mixture to low speed, to create a final stabilization of the foam before using.

COOKIES

Cookies are always welcome and do not need a lot of fanfare. They are essential for making the happy moments called ice cream sandwiches, which used to be my trick when I would notice someone having a rough day. A fresh sandwich would appear just for them, and all would be well again. Cookie dough is also a great place to play and freezes well, making way for freshly baked cookies in a pinch. The variations could be as simple as adding a spice or swapping of a kind of chocolate, resulting in a completely different cookie.

A cookie is often a great way to test out your baking skills. Use them to get to know your scale, learn to sift, and be mindful when baking—the only way to guarantee excellent sweet results. A cookie is only as good as its conception, including the temperature at which you give it life. Low baking temperatures will dry out cookies, whereas high temperatures will bake the outside, potentially leaving the inside raw. The goal is to find something right in the middle where a cookie achieves a touch of browning but still has a great texture from the sugar and fat inside the dough.

When I have strayed away from baking at times throughout the years, cookies always seem to bring me back to my mixer. I know that I will be able to accomplish the task with ease, and the results seem to have consistently reignited my affinity for both making and eating desserts. Think about it: after not having sweets for what may feel like way too long, sitting on a stoop having a great conversation with a straight-from-the-oven chocolate chip cookie. I have had this moment more than once and hope you will, too, with the gateway from Clean to Enough: freshly baked cookies.

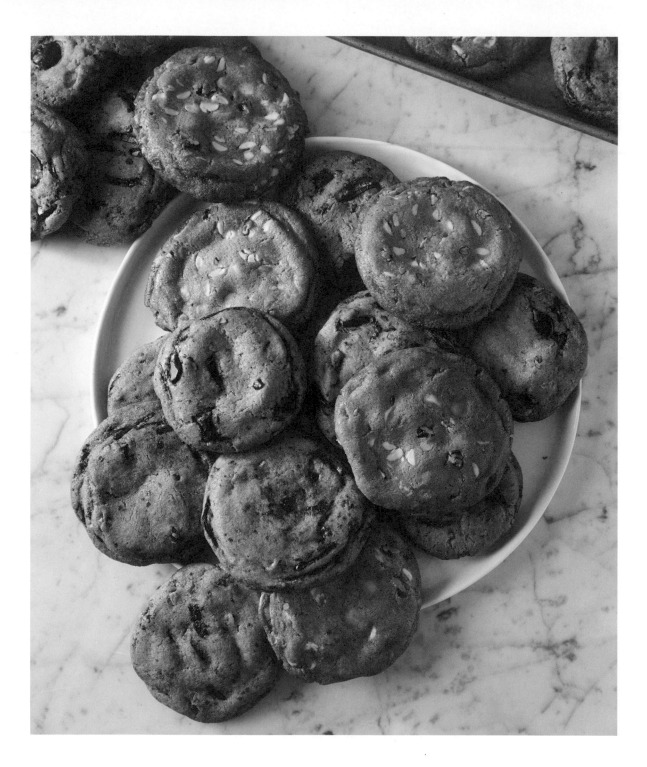

GENEROUS CHOCOLATE CHUNK COOKIES

There are a lot of opinions on what makes a great chocolate chip cookie. Over time, I've found my perfect bite in these Generous Chocolate Chunk Cookies. They are packed to the brim, well salted to offset the chocolate and sugary dough, and as easy to share as to devour solo. Hearty and not at all cakey. Girth over svelte. Perfected by a smattering of butter-loving toasted pecans.

Makes 34 cookies

¾ pound (3 sticks) + 2 tablespoons (360 g) unsalted organic butter, chilled and chopped into ½-inch (13 mm) chunks

1¾ cups + 1½ tablespoons (400 g) organic granulated cane sugar

1½ cups (320 g) packed light brown sugar

3½ large pasture-raised eggs (about 6½ ounces/180 g)

2½ teaspoons pure vanilla extract

2 teaspoons Maldon large flake sea salt

5 cups + 3 tablespoons (700 g) organic unbleached all-purpose flour

2¼ teaspoons baking soda

19½ ounces (550 g) 70% dark chocolate wafers (Michel Cluizel preferred)

1 heaping cup (125 g) pecans, lightly toasted and roughly chopped

1. Preheat the oven to 325°F (165°C) convection and line a half sheet pan with parchment paper.

2. Combine the butter chunks with the granulated and brown sugars in a stand mixer fitted with the paddle attachment. Start the mixer on low speed to break down the butter with the sugars. Increase the speed to high and cream the butter with the sugars for 7 minutes, or until the mixture is fluffy and light in color because of the air incorporated. Scrape down the sides of the bowl, using a rubber spatula, being sure to get to the bottom.

3. With the mixer running on medium speed, combine the eggs, one at a time, with the butter mixture and beat in the vanilla. Scrape down the sides and bottom of the bowl. Add the sea salt and mix for a few seconds to combine.

4. Sift the flour with the baking soda two times until any clumps are gone. Add to the butter mixture and mix on low speed until evenly blended. Scrape down the bowl again, ensuring no butter chunks remain.

5. Add the chocolate wafers and roughly chopped pecans to the batter. Paddle the mixture on low speed, to just incorporate the chocolate.

6. Scoop the dough into heaping ¼-cup (50 g) balls and place on the prepared half sheet pan, eight to a pan.

7. Bake for 15 minutes. Then turn the pan of cookies and bake for an additional 4 to 6 minutes, until just golden around the edges and no longer wet in the center.

8. Transfer the cookies to a cooling rack to cool for about 15 minutes. When cooled, store in an airtight container at room temperature.

WHITE CHOCOLATE MOLASSES COOKIES

The chewy spicy bite of a great molasses cookie, ripe with spices and cut with creamy and sweet, slightly caramelized white chocolate chunks: heaven. Use blackstrap molasses for the biggest punch; a good dark organic molasses or black treacle will also do the trick. These cookies reflect my acquired taste for Syrian pepper—a combination of sweet spices and black pepper that we used as a go-to seasoning for meats and stews (and these cookies) when I was growing up.

These cookies are better the next day, in my opinion, letting the spices and sugars settle. Want another trade secret? Sandwich two with a scoop of vanilla custard and a scoop of the apple pie filling from the Caramelized Apple Pie recipe (page 172) in between for pie crossed with an ice cream sandwich.

Makes 16 cookies

12 tablespoons (1½ sticks/170 g) unsalted organic butter, chilled and chopped into ½-inch (13 mm) chunks

¾ cup + 2 tablespoons (175 g) packed light brown sugar

⅓ cup (100 g) blackstrap molasses

¾ teaspoon ground ginger

½ teaspoon ground Ceylon cinnamon

¼ teaspoon freshly grated nutmeg

¼ teaspoon freshly ground black pepper

⅛ teaspoon ground cloves

⅛ teaspoon ground allspice

1 large pasture-raised egg (50 g)

2½ teaspoons pure vanilla extract

1¾ cups + 1½ tablespoons (250 g) organic unbleached all-purpose flour

½ teaspoon baking soda

¼ teaspoon fine sea salt

5½ ounces (160 g) white chocolate wafers (Michel Cluizel preferred)

Organic granulated cane sugar for rolling

1. Preheat the oven to 325°F (165°C) convection and line a half sheet pan with parchment paper.

2. Combine the butter with the brown sugar, molasses, ginger, cinnamon, nutmeg, pepper, cloves, and allspice in a stand mixer fitted with the paddle attachment. Start the mixer on low speed to break down the butter with the sugar. Increase the speed to high and mix for 1 minute. Scrape down the sides and bottom of the bowl.

3. Add the egg and vanilla to the butter mixture and blend for 3 minutes. Scrape down the sides and bottom of the bowl.

4. Sift the all-purpose flour with the baking soda and salt two times. Add to the butter mixture and mix on low speed until evenly combined. Scrape down the bowl again, ensuring no butter chunks remain.

5. Add the chocolate wafers to the batter. Paddle to just incorporate.

6. Scoop the dough into heaping ¼-cup (50 g) balls and place them on the prepared half sheet pan, eight to a pan. For a more rounded cookie, chill the dough in the refrigerator for 10 to 20 minutes.

7. Roll the cookie dough balls in granulated sugar, then bake for 12 minutes.

8. Turn the pan of cookies and bake for an additional 5 to 7 minutes, until just golden around the edges and no longer wet in the center.

9. Transfer the cookies to a cooling rack to cool for about 15 minutes. When cooled, store in an airtight container at room temperature, or throw them in the fridge to have ready for fresh ice cream sandwiches.

TEA RAISIN OATMEAL COOKIES

I have always said that New England bohemians—read: hippies—make the best oatmeal raisin cookies. Why? Because they are usually chock-full of oats. I like my oatmeal raisin cookies to be hearty and these fit the bill. Plumped dried fruit is always an excellent opportunity to add additional flavor to a recipe by fattening the fruit into something unique. Raisins soaked in tea is my favorite way to plump the fruit, adding pops of flavor to an already flavorful cookie.

Makes 16 cookies

½ pound (2 sticks/225 g) unsalted organic butter, chilled and chopped into ½-inch (13 mm) chunks

1 cup (215 g) organic granulated cane sugar

½ cup + 1 tablespoon (125 g) packed light brown sugar

2 tablespoons blackstrap molasses

½ teaspoon ground Ceylon cinnamon

½ teaspoon freshly ground nutmeg

½ teaspoon fresh orange zest

2 large pasture-raised eggs (100 g)

1 teaspoon pure vanilla extract

1 cup (135 g) organic unbleached all-purpose flour

1¼ teaspoons baking soda

½ teaspoon fine sea salt

3 cups (280 g) thick-cut rolled oats (Bob's Red Mill preferred)

¾ cup (65 g) ground oats

½ cup (80 g) Chamomile Raisins (page 243), soaked and squeezed

½ cup (80 g) Earl Grey Raisins (page 243), soaked and squeezed

½ cup (50 g) unsweetened desiccated coconut

1. Combine the butter with the granulated and brown sugars, molasses, cinnamon, nutmeg, and zest in a stand mixer fitted with the paddle attachment.

2. Start the mixer on low speed to break down the butter with the sugar. Increase the speed to high and cream the butter with the sugars for 5 minutes. Scrape down, using a rubber spatula, being sure to scrape the bottom of the bowl.

3. Add the eggs, one at a time, to the butter mixture and beat in the vanilla. Scrape down the sides and bottom of the bowl.

4. Sift the all-purpose flour with baking soda and salt two times, then whisk in the rolled oats and oat flour. Add the flour mixture to the butter mixture and mix on low speed until evenly combined.

5. Add the raisins and coconut to the batter. Scrape down the bowl again, ensuring no butter chunks remain. Paddle to just combine.

6. Scoop the dough into heaping ¼-cup (50 g) balls, and place them on a parchment-lined half sheet pan, eight to a pan. Chill the dough in the fridge for 30 minutes before baking to prevent excess spreading.

7. Twenty minutes before you bake, preheat the oven to 325°F (165°C) convection.

8. Bake the chilled cookies in the oven for 10 minutes.

9. Turn the pan of cookies and bake for an additional 5 minutes, or until just golden around the edges and no longer wet in the center.

10. Transfer the cookies to a cooling rack to cool for about 15 minutes. When cooled, store in an airtight container at room temperature, or throw them in the fridge to have ready for fresh ice cream sandwiches.

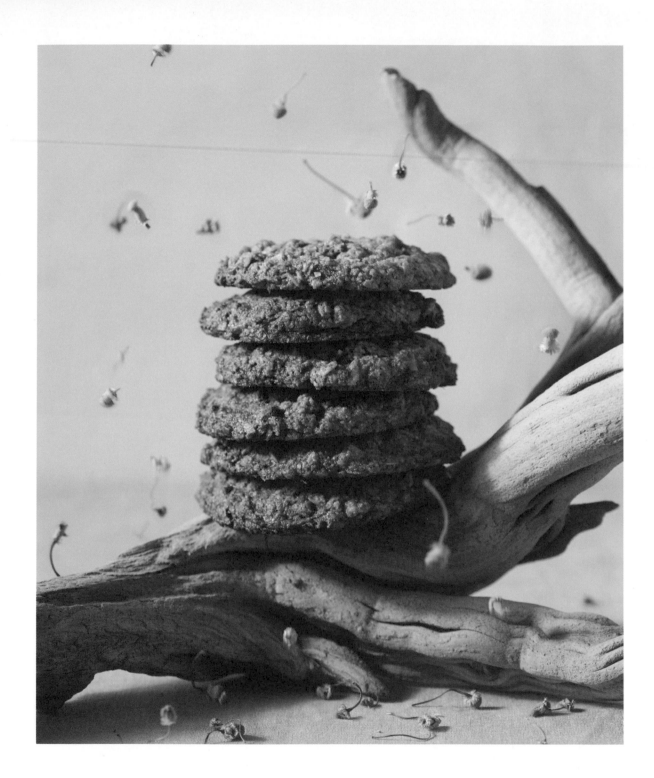

SHORTBREAD SERIES

The base recipe of these little drops of pure butter love can be used for a multitude of cookies, whether filled, thumbprints, made nuttier with whole wheat flour, or rolled into a piecrust. Swap in brown rice and whole wheat flours? You have a Digestive Biscuit, a nutty staple I grew up eating in Canada. Fill with fig and pineapple puree? Better than a Fig Newton. Rolled in vanilla sugar? Droplets of afternoon tea happiness. Flattened into disks to be filled with honey butter and dipped in meringue? Bianca is the word for these pure white sandwich cookies; the holy grail of the shortbread series, they are inspired by *alfajores* that I enjoyed for the first time walking through the old city in Jerusalem.

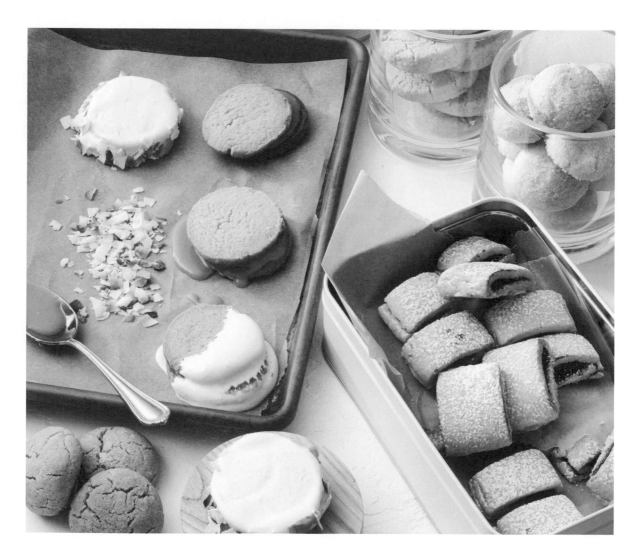

CLASSIC SHORTBREAD

Makes 35 cookies

VANILLA SUGAR

Scant ½ cup (100 g) organic
  granulated cane sugar

½ vanilla bean pod (with or without
  seeds still intact)

DOUGH

¾ pound (3 sticks) + 1 tablespoon
  (350 g) unsalted organic butter,
  chilled and cut into ½-inch (13 mm)
  chunks

3¼ cups (400 g) pastry flour (see
  Notes)

⅔ cup + ½ tablespoon (150 g) organic
  granulated cane sugar

⅓ cup (50 g) rice flour (see Notes)

¼ cup + 2 tablespoons (50 g)
  confectioners' sugar

Pinch of fine sea salt

1. To make the vanilla sugar, place the sugar and vanilla bean in a food processor and grind to combine. Store in an airtight container.

2. To make the cookie dough, combine all the dough ingredients in a stand mixer fitted with the paddle attachment. Start the mixer on low speed to break down the butter with the sugar. Increase the speed to medium and continue to paddle the dough until the dough becomes crumbly and then begins to come together into a homogenous mixture.

3. Divide and shape the dough into two equal square packs and wrap with plastic wrap. Chill in the fridge for 1 hour.

4. Preheat the oven to 325°F (165°C) convection and line a half sheet pan with parchment.

5. To make shortbread drops, portion the dough into heaping 2-tablespoon balls. Roll the cookies in the vanilla sugar and place on the prepared half sheet pan, 1 inch (2.5 cm) apart.

6. Bake the shortbread for 10 minutes. Then turn the pan and bake for an additional 2 to 6 minutes, until just golden around the edges and still very pale and snow white.

7. Remove the cookies from the oven and dust with additional vanilla sugar.

8. Allow the cookies to cool on the pan and then store in an airtight container at room temperature.

NOTES

The vanilla in the rolling sugar can easily be replaced by ½ teaspoon lavender, rosemary, lemon zest, or another aromatic that you love.

When freezing dough for future baking, roll the cookies in vanilla sugar first.

Pastry flour is finer than all-purpose flour. If you only have all-purpose you can replace ¼ cup (30 g) flour with cornstarch.

I often place white jasmine rice in a dry high-speed blender and grind instead of buying rice flour. This results in a slightly different, more textured shortbread mixture of butter, rice, and sugar.

DIGESTIVE BISCUIT

Makes 30 cookies

¾ pound (3 sticks) + 1 tablespoon (350 g) unsalted organic butter, chilled and cut into ½-inch (13 mm) chunks

3¼ cups (400 g) whole wheat pastry flour

¾ cup (150 g) granulated demerara sugar, plus more for rolling

⅓ cup (50 g) brown rice flour

¼ cup + 2 tablespoons (50 g) confectioners' sugar

¼ teaspoon ground Ceylon cinnamon

Pinch of fine sea salt

1. Combine all the ingredients in a stand mixer fitted with the paddle attachment.

2. Start the mixer on low speed to break down the butter with the sugar. Increase the speed to medium and continue to paddle the dough until it becomes crumbly and then begins to come together into a homogenous mixture.

3. Divide and shape the dough into two equal square packs and wrap with plastic wrap. Roll the dough into two logs about 10 inches (25.5 cm) long each.

4. Roll the logs in demerara sugar, then wrap in parchment or plastic wrap and chill in the fridge for 1 hour.

5. Preheat the oven to 325°F (165°C) convection and line a half sheet pan with parchment.

6. Using a standard kitchen knife, cut the chilled cookie logs into slices about ¼ to ½ inch (6 mm to 13 mm) thick. Place the slices on the prepared half sheet pan, 1 inch (2.5 cm) apart.

7. Bake for 10 minutes, then turn the pan of cookies and bake for an additional 4 to 6 minutes, until slightly browned around the edges.

8. Remove the cookies from the oven and allow to cool on the pan. Store in an airtight container at room temperature.

FIGGY NEWTONS

Makes 20 cookies

1 cup (175 g) dried figs

⅓ cup + 1 tablespoon (95 ml)
  pineapple juice

1 teaspoon grated fresh ginger

½ batch Classic Shortbread dough
  (page 142)

All-purpose flour for rolling pin

Confectioners' sugar for dusting

1. Using kitchen scissors, stem the figs and snip them in half. Place in a food processor.

2. Warm the pineapple juice and ginger in a small saucepan over medium heat and pour over the dried figs. Puree until smooth. Cool the mixture in the fridge for 15 minutes, or until ready to bake.

3. Take a roughly 8½-ounce (250 g) portion of shortbread dough and place on a piece of parchment on the countertop. Using a floured rolling pin, hit the dough to soften the butter slightly. Roll the shortbread into a 5 x 11-inch (12.5 x 28 cm) rectangle.

4. Spread a 1½-inch (4 cm)-thick line of fig filling down the center of the rectangle. Starting from the bottom, fold up the dough, using the parchment to help encase the filling and meet the other side of the dough. Allow the two ends of dough to overlap slightly so that no fig filling leaks out. Pat gently to seal the shortbread dough together.

5. Wrap the filled dough completely in the parchment and chill it on a sheet pan for 30 minutes.

6. Meanwhile, preheat the oven to 325°F (165°C) convection and line a half sheet pan with parchment paper.

7. Remove the dough from the fridge and slice the log into 1½-inch (4 cm) pieces. Place on the prepared half sheet pan. Bake for 10 minutes, then turn the pan of cookies and bake for 6 minutes more, until slightly golden around the edges.

8. Remove the cookies from the oven and dust generously with confectioners' sugar.

9. Allow the cookies to cool on the pan and then store in an airtight container at room temperature.

NOTE

You can easily roll balls of shortbread dough and create thumbprints to fill with fig filling before baking instead of creating a filled cookie.

BIANCAS

Makes 20 cookies

1 batch Classic Shortbread dough
(page 142)

1 cup (225 g) Honey Butter (page
239)

1 recipe Swiss Meringue (page 206),
prepared through step 8

Pinch of ground Ceylon cinnamon

1 cup (75 g) toasted coconut flakes
(see Notes)

1. Roll out the chilled shortbread dough to ¼ inch (6 mm) thick on a piece of parchment paper. Cut the dough into circles 2 inches (5 cm) in diameter. Place the cookies on a parchment-lined half sheet pan and place in the freezer for at least 15 minutes.

2. Meanwhile, preheat the oven to 325°F (165°C) convection.

3. Bake the cookies until just golden around the edges, about 15 minutes. Remove the cookies from the oven and allow to cool on the pan.

4. Sandwich two cooled cookies together with 1 teaspoon of the Honey Butter. Repeat with the remaining cookies. Return the cookies to the fridge.

5. Whip the meringue until it reaches soft peaks; add the cinnamon.

6. Set up a fresh half sheet pan lined with parchment and a shallow plate of coconut flakes next to the bowl of meringue. Preheat the oven to 200°F (95°C) convection.

7. Remove the cookies from the fridge. Using a small offset spatula or spoon, spread a heaping double-tablespoon dollop of meringue over each entire sandwich cookie (top, sides, and bottom), covering it completely. You will get meringue on your hands—this is okay!

8. Roll the edges of the meringue-coated cookies in toasted coconut flakes and carefully place on the prepared half sheet pan. At this point you can smooth out the top of the meringue with your spoon or spatula.

9. Place the coated meringue cookies in the oven to dry out the meringue, 90 minutes, turning the pan after about 60 minutes, to ensure even drying.

10. When cooled on the pan, store at room temperature in an airtight container.

NOTES

Toast coconut flakes at 300°F (150°C) in a single layer on a sheet pan. Keep your eye on the coconut flakes as they burn easily.

If the meringue is fully whipped before you are ready to coat the cookie sandwiches, lower the stand mixer to its lowest speed, which will keep the meringue stable without whipping it further.

CANTUCCINI

The first time I had a cantuccini, it was perched atop a glass of *vino santo*. I was at a loud restaurant in Florence, where I had taken the train from Milan, just for dinner. I will remember that amazing day for the rest of my life, because it captured the essence of me: a perfect meal, a dainty sweet bite, and life's simple, adventurous pleasures, all embodied in this humble cookie. They are perfect alone or with coffee, sweet wine, a scoop of vanilla custard, or Whipped Cream Glacé (page 221)—and always a big smile.

Makes 24 cookies

⅔ cup + ½ tablespoon (150 g) organic granulated cane sugar

¼ cup (50 g) packed light brown sugar

Scant ¼ cup (55 ml) extra virgin olive oil

1 large pasture-raised egg (50 g)

1 large pasture-raised egg yolk (20 g)

½ teaspoon ground Ceylon cinnamon

¼ teaspoon ground anise

⅛ teaspoon freshly grated nutmeg

2 cups (250 g) whole wheat pastry flour

½ teaspoon baking powder

Pinch of salt

½ cup (7 g) pine nuts, untoasted

1. Combine the granulated and brown sugars with the olive oil, egg and egg yolk, and spices in a stand mixer fitted with the whisk attachment. Whip on medium speed until the sugar is dissolved, about 5 minutes.

2. Sift the flour with the baking powder and salt into a bowl. Fold the nuts into flour, then fold the flour mixture into the egg mixture.

3. Line two half sheet pans with parchment. Pat the dough into two logs, each about 4 inches (10 cm) wide and the length of a half sheet pan on a diagonal. Place one log on each prepared half sheet pan. Place the pans in the fridge for 15 minutes.

4. Meanwhile, preheat the oven to 325°F (165°C) convection. Bake the whole cantuccini logs for 10 minutes, then turn the pans and bake for an additional 10 minutes, until slightly golden but still pale.

5. Allow the cookie logs to cool on the pan for 15 minutes for easier slicing. Then, using a serrated knife, cut the cookies into ¼- to ½-inch (6 mm to 13 mm) slices, laying them flat on their pans in rows, twelve per sheet.

6. Return the cookies to the oven to bake for 10 minutes, then turn the pans and bake for an additional 7 to 10 minutes, to fully crisp. Allow the cantuccini to cool on a wire rack and then store in an airtight container.

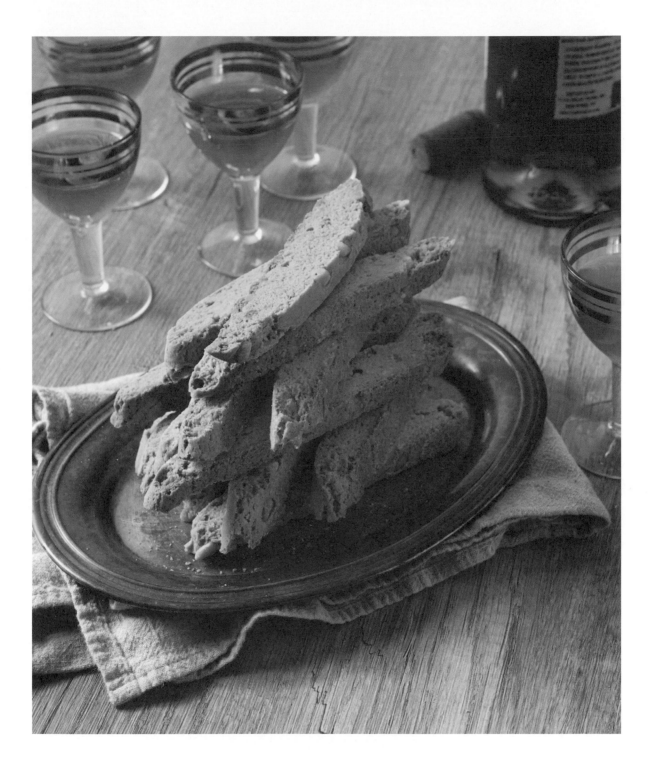

ROASTED COCONUT COOKIES

Oh, to roast coconut. It's a far more seductive approach than mere toasting, as roasting is done slowly at a lower temperature. I have burned many pans of coconut flakes in my lifetime by placing the dried meat in a too-hot oven. This rich chocolate cookie has seen many variations, the best one being when all flours—wheat, chickpea, or otherwise—did not make their way into the mixing bowl. The large amount of roasted coconut is all that holds this cookie together, apart from its generous addition of dark chocolate. This cookie was inspired by my favorite praline from Max Brenner Chocolate Bar, which was full of roasted coconut and perfectly smooth ganache, a study in textures. The attention to detail needed to create the right flavor profile of coconut *before* folding it into rich chocolate cream has always stuck with me: Handle with care!

Makes 2 dozen cookies

3 cups (250 g) large flake unsweetened coconut

11 ounces (320 g) 70% dark chocolate wafers (Michel Cluizel preferred)

1¼ cups (280 g) packed light brown sugar

4 tablespoons (55 g) organic unsalted butter, softened and pliable

1 teaspoon baking powder

3 large pasture-raised eggs (150 g)

1 teaspoon pure vanilla extract

¼ teaspoon Maldon sea salt flakes

1. Preheat the oven to 300°F (150°C) convection and line a half sheet pan with parchment.

2. Place the coconut flakes in a single layer on the prepared half sheet pan and roast, stirring every few minutes, until evenly golden, about 15 minutes. Once the coconut has roasted, remove from the oven, increase the oven temperature to 325°F (165°C) convection, and line a second half sheet pan with parchment.

3. Meanwhile, place the chocolate in a medium glass bowl and microwave for 1 minute. Stir and continue to microwave the chocolate at 30-second intervals until it is melted and warm but not too hot.

4. Place the sugar, butter, and baking powder in a stand mixer fitted with the paddle attachment. Blend on high speed for 3 minutes.

5. Stream in the melted chocolate and continue to paddle for 3 minutes. Scrape down the bowl and add the eggs, one at a time, and vanilla. Fold in the roasted coconut and salt.

6. Place ¼-cup (50 g) scoops of batter on the prepared second half sheet pan, 1 inch (2.5 cm) apart. Because the batter is full of chocolate, it may firm up. If the batter hardens, roll the cookies slightly and place them back on the cookie pan, flattening slightly with the palm of your hand.

7. Bake for 8 minutes, then turn the pan of cookies and bake for an additional 4 to 5 minutes, until no longer wet looking on the top. Allow the cookies to cool on a wire rack and then store in an airtight container. They are also excellent rewarmed, as warming softens the chocolate and amplifies the coconut flavor.

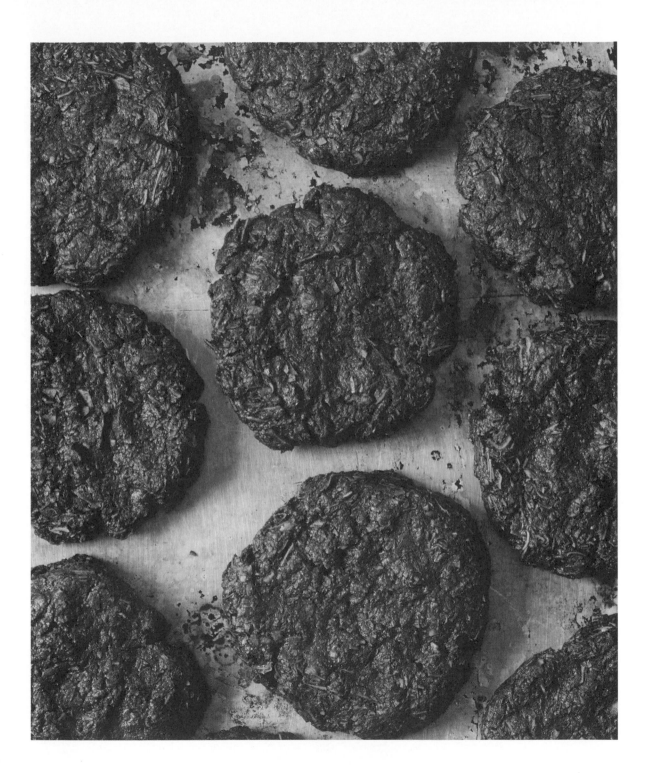

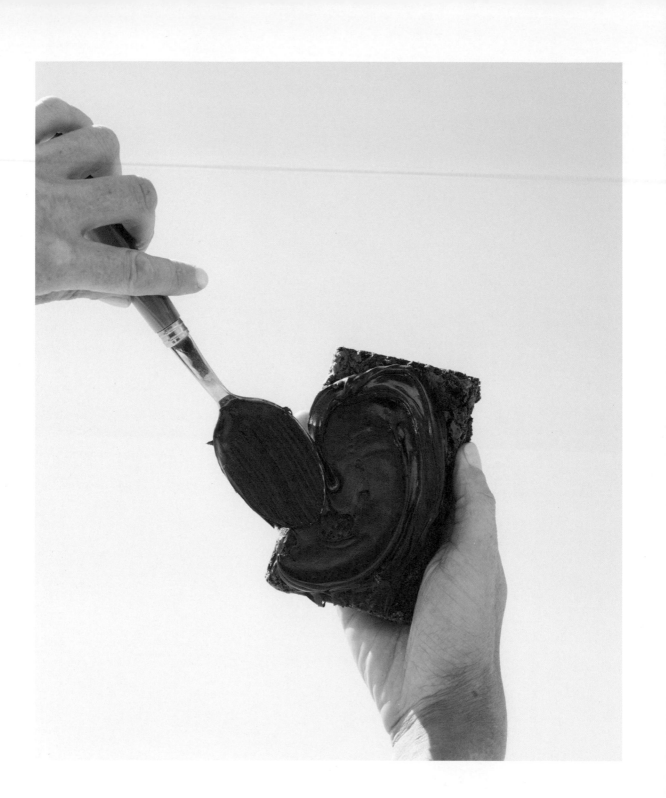

BROWNIES WITH A SCHMEAR

These brownies are rich, fudgy, and almost exclusively pure chocolate with a smattering of cocoa powder in the batter, whereas most brownie recipes rely primarily on cocoa powder. The best part of these brownies is the schmear. What is a schmear? Imagine the perfect bagel with just enough cream cheese. For a chocolate schmear, take big spoonsful of chocolate ganache, or rich chocolate hazelnut cream, and spread on top of the brownie in an S shape, using the back of the spoon.

Makes 1 quarter sheet pan of brownies (9 x 13 inches/23 x 33 cm)

Nonstick spray

9½ ounces (275 g) 70% dark chocolate wafers (Michel Cluizel preferred)

½ pound (2 sticks/225 g) unsalted organic butter, softened and pliable

3 large pasture-raised eggs (150 g)

¾ cup + 2 tablespoons (200 g) organic granulated cane sugar

¼ cup (50 g) packed light brown sugar

1 tablespoon + 1 teaspoon pure vanilla extract

1½ teaspoons fine sea salt

¼ cup (25 g) unsweetened cocoa powder

1 cup + 2 tablespoons (150 g) organic unbleached all-purpose flour

1½ teaspoons (5 g) baking powder

3½ ounces (100 g) milk chocolate wafers (Michel Cluizel preferred)

1. Preheat the oven to 250°F (120°C) convection. Line a quarter sheet pan with parchment and spray with nonstick spray.

2. Place the 70% chocolate in a glass bowl in the microwave or in a bowl set over simmering water and melt until warm but not too hot. Add the butter and stir to combine.

3. Combine the eggs, granulated and brown sugars, cocoa powder, vanilla, and salt in a stand mixer fitted with the whisk attachment. Whisk on high speed for 3 minutes to dissolve the sugar without aerating the mixture. Add the melted chocolate to the eggs and mix to combine fully, without whipping, about 1 minute.

4. Sift together the flour and baking powder. Add the flour mixture to the chocolate mixture and whisk to just combine. Roughly chop the milk chocolate and fold it into the chocolate mixture. Pour the brownie batter into the prepared pan.

5. Bake for 15 minutes, then turn the pan and bake for 5 minutes, or until fully baked in the center but not dry.

NOTES

This recipe can be made by hand, without using a stand mixer. Simply whisk the egg mixture together in a large bowl for 4 to 5 minutes, until the sugar is dissolved.

Some people love baking brownies in a Pyrex glass baking dish. This is totally doable, but if you do, I recommend using an 8-inch (20.5 cm) square dish.

Add a ½ cup (115 ml) swirl of Original Treacle Sauce (page 234) to the finished batter to take these to the next level!

CAKE!

I have found that people start out in two camps when it comes to cake: for or against. Dry, bland wedding cake slivers or office party cakes with the faux, fatty frosting must have really left a negative mark on the world, for cake can and should be a celebratory dish or fantastic slice with an afternoon tea or coffee. Cake does not need to be dry, unless of course you overcook it. Cake does not need to be flavorless when it can include high-quality vanilla, citrus zests, grated vegetables, fruit, or dangerously dark cocoa. Cake frosting, well, that can often take the cake! From deeply dense and dark milky dark frosting or bright and creamy whipped mascarpone to glossy lime meringue, every flavor and color deserves their time to shine.

Cake is a level up from the cookie game, requiring precise measuring (on your scale); proper sifting of dry ingredients, ensuring no clumps; gentle mixing; and, of course, proper pan preparation and baking. Do not forget the patience required when cooling! Cakes should cool on their own at room temperature, ensuring that the crumb structure created stays intact. A cooled cake will always slice more easily, allowing you to fill and frost as you please.

I have a thing for casual approachability even when it comes to cake assembly. Mile-high tiered cakes can be intimidating to the home baker and even the eater, and while I love the unmasked, frosting-free cakes, showing the individual layers, as well as cakes adorned with drips, drizzles, and a multitude of toppings, I truly love low, flat, round cakes and tortes. Serve them simply on a beautiful flat platter, no pomp and circumstance, just effortless beauty and yum. You will find all of the cakes to be single-tier frosted or bare or, at most, split in half, filled with something flavorful and pungent, masked with anything from chocolate, cream, meringue, or whipped cream cheese.

Cakes are true gifts; make them to celebrate someone, something, or you.

COCONUT CAKE WITH TOASTED LIME MERINGUE

This cake happened by accident. I needed to assemble the Easter dessert for our then restaurant at the Grand Hyatt on the fly. I whipped up a batch of a great birthday cake recipe and saw a pineapple out of the corner of my eye. I thought, *when in Rome*, so chunks of the pineapple along with some untoasted coconut went right into the batter. I wanted to frost this cake with cream cheese frosting, as most coconut cakes should be. I started stacking the layers and thought, *I don't want this cake to taste flat; let's add some lemon curd and* toasted *coconut to the filling*. Then I realized I had not made enough frosting to top the large sheet cake. One of the pastry cooks, Eve, was whipping a batch of lime meringue for clouds, which quickly was repositioned as a luscious top layer of lime meringue on the cake. Cut into perfect squares and toasted to order, this cake became the special order for all birthdays and celebrations, including my best friend's multitiered wedding cake adorned with delicate hydrangea many years later.

Makes 10 to 12 servings

Nonstick spray or softened butter for pan

13 tablespoons (1 stick + 5 tablespoons/180 g) organic unsalted butter, softened and pliable

1¾ + 1½ tablespoons (400 g) organic granulated cane sugar

1 ounce (30 g) white chocolate wafers, (Michel Cluizel preferred)

4 large pasture-raised eggs (200 g), separated

Scant 1 cup (220 ml/225 g) organic buttermilk

1 teaspoon pure vanilla extract

2 cups (280 g) organic unbleached all-purpose flour

1 teaspoon baking powder

¼ teaspoon fine sea salt

½ cup (100 g) finely chopped fresh pineapple

½ cup (40 g) desiccated coconut, untoasted

1. Preheat the oven to 325°F (165°C) convection. Line an 11-inch (28 cm) round springform pan with a parchment round, coated with nonstick spray.

2. Combine the softened butter with 1¾ cups (350 g) of the granulated sugar in a stand mixer fitted with the paddle attachment. Whip on high speed for 5 minutes.

3. Meanwhile, melt the white chocolate in a bowl in the microwave, or in a bowl on top of a pot of simmering water. Scrape the bowl down. Scoop a small portion (about ½ cup/100 g) of the butter mixture and stir into the warm melted white chocolate.

4. Add the white chocolate mixture to the mixer and mix on high speed to combine. Add the egg yolks, mixing them in and scraping down the sides of the bowl.

5. Add half of the buttermilk and the vanilla to the batter; whip to combine.

6. Sift the flour with the baking powder and salt. Add half of the flour mixture to the mixer. Scrape the bowl well and add the remaining buttermilk while running the mixer on medium speed. Add the remaining flour, scraping down the sides of the bowl. Fold in the pineapple and untoasted coconut.

recipe continues . . .

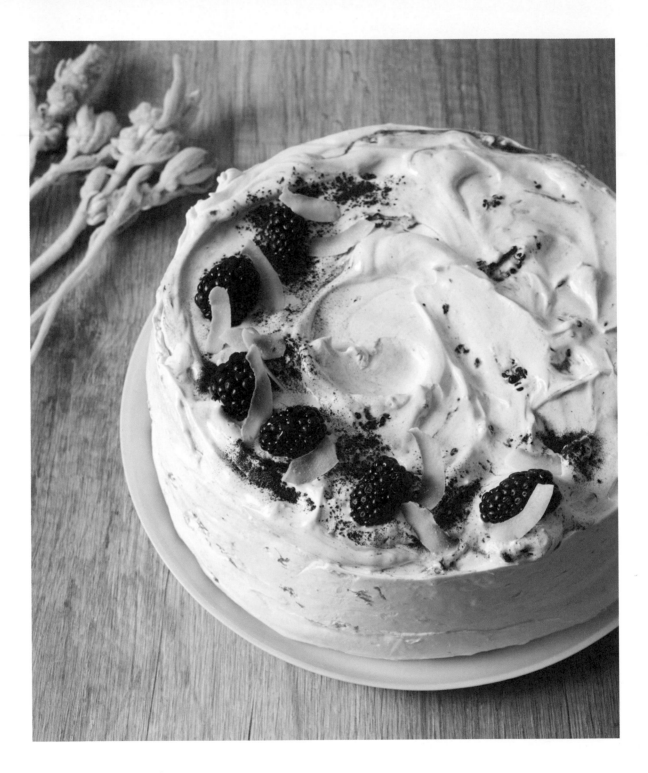

TO ASSEMBLE

1 cup (225 g) Cream Cheese Frosting (page 240)

¾ cup (175 g) Creamy Lemon Curd (page 242)

½ to 1 pint (150 to 300 g) blackberries, optional

3 cups (300 g) Lime Clouds meringue (page 208), whipped to stiff peaks

1 cup (80 g) unsweetened desiccated coconut, toasted, plus more for decorating

The very original recipe for this cake batter, unmasked and altered, was taught to me by Sherry Yard, my mentor, friend, and pastry trailblazer. Sherry learned it from Sixto Pocasangre, her right hand who headed up Wolfgang Puck Catering, making its way into her second book, *Desserts by the Yard*. This sticky, sweet, delicious cake was always on hand at Spago, where we were given a moment's notice to produce a birthday cake, which is all we needed! Adding white chocolate to the cake batter in this recipe is utter genius: It solves all issues related to the moisture and sweet vanilla flavor of boxed cake that many people were brought up on.

7. Whip the egg whites by hand in a clean metal bowl, using a large balloon whisk or the largest whisk that you have, as this will making whipping your whites easier. When the egg whites begin to foam, sprinkle in the remaining ¼ cup (50 g) of sugar slowly, while whipping.

8. Once the egg whites have formed glossy soft peaks, add a small scoop of the whites to the cake batter to lighten it without deflating the entire batch of whites. Then add the remaining beaten whites to the cake batter and fold gently to combine. Pour the batter into the prepared pan.

9. Bake the cake for 30 to 40 minutes, until golden, turning the pan halfway through that time to ensure even baking.

10. Remove the cake from the oven and allow to cool before releasing the sides of the springform pan, about an hour. Place the cake in the freezer for another hour. This will make it easier to slice the cake in half to fill.

11. To assemble: Place the cake on a platter or cake stand and carefully slice in half horizontally, using a long, serrated knife.

12. Spread a generous even layer of Cream Cheese Frosting onto the bottom round of cake. Spread a generous even layer of Creamy Lemon Curd on top of the cream cheese frosting. Stud the blackberries, if using, on top of the lemon curd and sprinkle with the toasted coconut flakes. Carefully place the top cake round on top.

13. Pile the top of the cake with Lime Clouds meringue. Begin spreading the meringue on the top of the cake, working your way down the sides. Use a small offset spatula to create swirls and peaks of the meringue. Have fun! The cake should look playful.

14. Turn on the broiler and set your oven rack in the center of the oven. Place the cake under the broiler briefly to toast the top of the cake. Alternatively, you can use a kitchen blowtorch to gently toast the top of the cake.

15. Decorate the top of the cake with additional roasted coconut flakes and blackberries, if desired.

16. Serve the cake in slices at room temperature. Store leftover cake, covered, in the refrigerator for up to a week.

PAN DI SPAGNA

This cake evokes effortless elegance. *Pan di spagna* equates to "sponge cake" in Italian, and what it soaks up is lemon syrup, before being filled with freshly whipped Mascarpone Cream, a bit of Creamy Lemon Curd, and a bounty of fresh fruit and nuts. I first made this cake for a gorgeous wedding at an estate in upstate New York: a 36 inch (92 cm) single tier cake. It was quite a sight, and *almost* as elegant as the bride. From that moment I fell in love with this cake, the idea of this cake, making this cake, assembling this cake, and gifting this cake to a beaming couple in love. I know that this will be my wedding cake, as I want my friends to tuck into something so simple and fresh after a beautiful dinner full of love and good wine.

Makes 10 to 12 servings

Nonstick spray or softened butter
  for pan

6 large pasture-raised eggs (300 g),
  at room temperature

¾ cup + 2 tablespoons (200 g)
  organic granulated cane sugar

1 teaspoon grated lemon zest

1 teaspoon vanilla bean paste; 1 vanilla
  bean, scraped; or 2 teaspoons pure
  vanilla extract

2 tablespoons (30 g) organic unsalted
  butter, melted

1 tablespoon fresh lemon juice

1½ cups (200 g) cake flour

½ teaspoon fine sea salt

¼ teaspoon baking powder

LEMON SYRUP

Scant ¼ cup (50 grams) organic
  granulated cane sugar

1 teaspoon grated lemon zest

2 teaspoons fresh lemon juice

1. Preheat the oven to 325°F (165°C) convection. Line an 11-inch (30.5 cm) round springform pan with a parchment round, coated with nonstick spray or brushed with softened butter.

2. Combine the eggs, sugar, lemon zest, and vanilla in a stand mixer fitted with the whisk attachment. Place the bowl on top of a pot of simmering water for 5 minutes, or until just warmed but not hot. Return the bowl to the mixer base.

3. Whip the egg mixture on medium speed for 8 to 10 minutes, until the egg foam reaches the top of the bowl and stops climbing.

4. In a separate bowl, combine the melted butter and lemon juice. Using a large spatula, gently fold the butter mixture into the egg foam.

5. Sift the flour, salt, and baking powder two times. Gently sift the flour mixture a third time directly over the egg foam and fold carefully, using a large balloon whisk or large spatula to combine, so as to not deflate the foam. Gently pour the batter into the prepared springform pan.

6. Bake the cake for 35 to 40 minutes, until just evenly golden, turning halfway through that time to ensure even baking. Remove from the oven and allow the cake to cool before unmolding from the springform pan.

recipe continues . . .

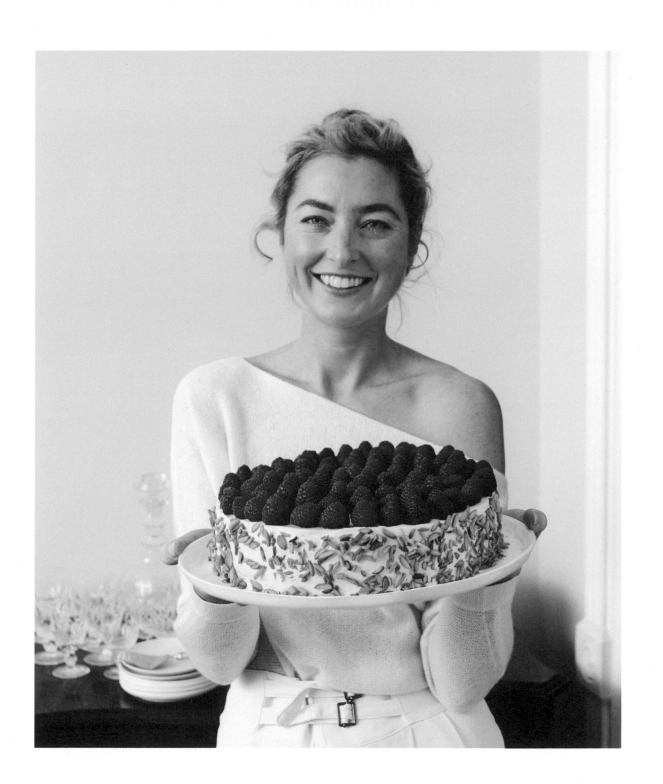

CAKE!

TO ASSEMBLE

3 pints (1 kg) baby strawberries or raspberries

½ cup (115 g) Creamy Lemon Curd (page 242)

2 batches Mascarpone Cream (page 245)

1 cup (125 g) raw Sicilian or regular pistachios, roughly chopped

7. To make the lemon syrup: Combine the sugar, 3 tablespoons (45 ml) water, and the lemon zest in a small saucepan and warm on medium heat to dissolve the sugar. Do not boil the syrup, as it will reduce the liquid. Whisk in the lemon juice.

8. To assemble: If using strawberries, remove the tops of the strawberries, inverting the berries, cut side down, on a paper towel–lined tray. If the strawberries are large, slice them into quarters lengthwise. Placing the cut berries on the paper towel will prevent the berries from bleeding onto the mascarpone. If using raspberries, leave whole.

9. Cut the cake round in half horizontally, using a long, serrated knife. Generously brush both sides of the cut cake layer with the lemon syrup.

10. Spread a thin layer of Creamy Lemon Curd over the bottom half of the cake. Spread 1 cup (225 g) Mascarpone Cream over the lemon curd. Stud the mascarpone cream with 1 cup (145 g) of the strawberries. Carefully place the second layer of the cake round on top.

11. Spread the remaining mascarpone first, working your way down the sides of the cake.

12. Coat the sides of the cake with the roughly chopped pistachios, by patting handfuls of the nuts along the sides of the cake, letting the excess fall onto a plate or parchment paper to catch them.

13. Cover the top of the cake completely with the remaining strawberries. The less cream in sight the better, as the top of the cake should be all fruit with the sides being all bright pistachios.

NOTES

This is a *very* simple cake that takes care and a delicate hand; be sure to sift the dry ingredients well and fold them into the batter gently, so as to not deflate the egg foam.

Do not overbake this cake! Once the cake is just golden and baked through, remove it from the oven. Simple sponge cakes like this can dry out easily.

Brush the cake generously with lemon syrup so that it is moist, without being soggy.

GRANDMA'S CHOCOLATE-CHOCOLATE-CHOCOLATE CAKE

This recipe is what I would refer to as "best of class." Sure it may seem like *just* a chocolate cake, albeit rich with cocoa and oil-based. But with the addition of brewed coffee, a great amount of dark cocoa, flaky sea salt, and ultra-rich chocolate bar frosting, the cake became next-level. It's good ever so slightly warmed from the oven, after the first chill in the fridge, or even pulled out of the freezer in a cake emergency.

Makes 10 servings

Nonstick spray or softened butter for pan

2 large pasture-raised eggs (100 g), at room temperature

Scant ¾ cup (150 g) organic granulated cane sugar

Scant ¾ cup (150 g) packed light brown sugar

½ cup + 2 tablespoons (150 ml) organic olive oil

⅓ cup (35 g) extra brut cocoa powder

¼ cup + 1 tablespoon (75 ml) hot brewed coffee

Scant ½ cup (110ml/115 g) organic buttermilk

½ teaspoon pure vanilla extract

1 cup + 2 tablespoons (150 g) organic unbleached all-purpose flour

1¼ teaspoons baking soda

¼ teaspoon fine sea salt

CHOCOLATE BAR FROSTING

8 ounces (225 g) 64% semisweet chocolate wafers (Michel Cluizel preferred)

Generous 2½ ounces (75 g) milk chocolate wafers (Michel Cluizel preferred)

1. Preheat the oven to 325°F (165°C) convection. Line an 11-inch (30.5 cm) round springform pan with a parchment round, coated with nonstick spray or brushed with softened butter.

2. Combine the eggs and granulated and brown sugars in a stand mixer fitted with the whisk attachment. Whip on high speed for 5 minutes to foam. Slowly stream in the oil with the mixer running on high speed, to combine thoroughly.

3. In a small bowl, whisk together the cocoa powder and coffee. Whisk in the buttermilk and vanilla. Add half of the cocoa mixture to the egg mixture. Whip to combine.

4. Sift the flour, baking soda, and salt. Add half of the flour mixture to the egg mixture. Mix to just combine. Add the remaining cocoa mixture, mix, and then add the remaining flour mixture.

5. Transfer the batter to the prepared pan and tap the pan on the counter to evenly distribute. As this is an oil-based cake batter that is fairly liquid, this is the easiest way to spread the batter evenly.

6. Bake for 35 to 45 minutes, rotating the pan halfway through that time to ensure even baking, until a toothpick inserted in the center of the cake comes out clean.

7. Remove the cake from the oven to cool completely before removing from the springform pan.

8. To make the frosting: Place the semisweet and milk chocolate in a glass bowl in the microwave or in a bowl on top of a pot of simmering water, and melt until warm but not too hot, about 1 minute in the microwave or 4 minutes on the stove. Stir together well to combine.

recipe continues . . .

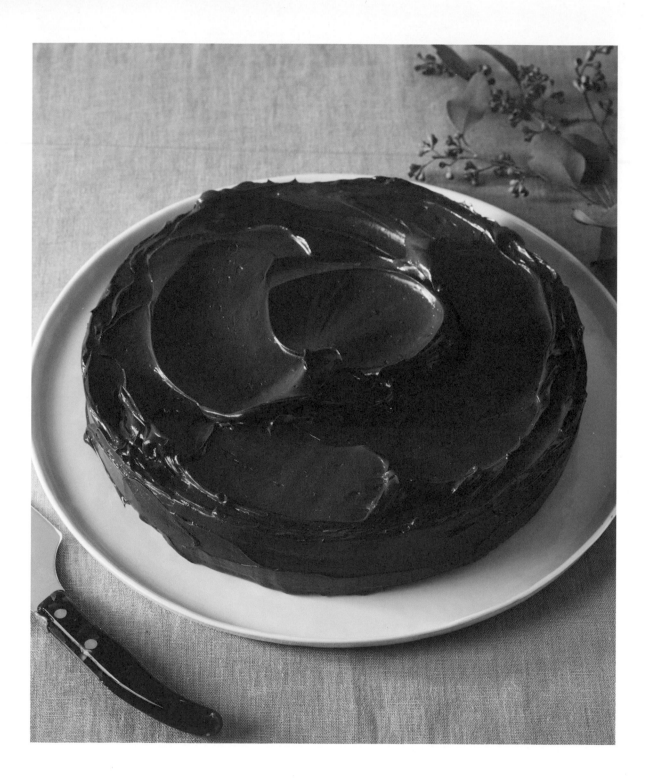

1 cup + 5 tablespoons (2 sticks + 5 tablespoons/300 g) organic unsalted butter, firm but at room temperature

½ teaspoon Maldon sea salt flakes, plus more for sprinkling

Crunchy chocolate pearls or sprinkles (optional)

9. Place the butter in a stand mixer fitted with the paddle attachment and mix on high speed for 4 minutes. Stream the melted chocolate into the butter while the mixer runs, scraping down the sides of the bowl as you go. Paddle in the salt.

10. To assemble, place the cake on a platter and split the cake round in half horizontally, using a long, serrated knife. Evenly spread 1½ cups (350 g) of the frosting on the bottom round of the cake. Carefully place the top round of the cake onto the frosted bottom layer. Place the remaining frosting on top of the cake and, using an offset spatula, spread the frosting evenly over the top and sides of the cake. The frosting can be as smooth or as rustic as you would like. Sprinkle the top of the cake with more Maldon sea salt flakes and crunchy chocolate pearls or sprinkles, if desired.

VARIATION

Raspberry Banana Chocolate Cake: Slice one banana into disks ¼ inch (6 mm) thick. After frosting the first layer of the cake, alternate banana slices with a pint (330 g) of fresh raspberries in a spiral beginning at the center of the cake round. Place the top cake round on top of the fruit, frost as usual, and then decorate the cake with fresh raspberries and crushed dried banana chips.

NOTE

If the frosting comes out too liquid, let it cool on the counter slightly or in the fridge until the sides begin to firm. Scrape down the sides of the bowl and place it back on the mixer stand, then whip with the paddle attachment to add air before frosting.

GARDEN CAKE

This carrot-beet cake is the divine base for which my infamous carrots were made on *Top Chef: Just Desserts*. We were tasked to create a world of pure imagination, and as a person who lives in my head, I built a garden of chocolate cookies and buried my carrots, with bowls of cream cheese icing tucked into pots in the garden. Children descended onto the set and were able to pick and play with their carrot patch. I have no idea how I thought of this: It must have been exhaustion, or maybe all pure imagination.

Since then, I've improved the recipe. With a smattering of cream cheese frosting (that grows in gardens, too, right?), toasted hazelnuts and fresh orange zest bring this cake to life. Keep it on hand for a taste of spring with your afternoon cup of tea.

Makes 10 servings

Nonstick spray or softened butter for pan

12 tablespoons (1½ sticks/180 g) unsalted organic butter, softened

¾ cup (160 g) organic granulated cane sugar

¼ cup (50 g) packed light brown sugar

1 teaspoon grated fresh ginger

1 teaspoon ground Ceylon cinnamon

¼ teaspoon grated orange zest

2 large pasture-raised eggs (100 g)

½ cup (60 g) hazelnuts, toasted and chopped, plus ½ cup (60 g) toasted and crushed

¾ cup (110 g) packed grated red beet (about 1 medium beet)

¾ cup (110 g) packed grated carrot (about 1 medium carrot)

¼ cup (30 g) diced pineapple

1½ cups (200 g) organic unbleached all-purpose flour

1 teaspoon baking soda

½ teaspoon baking powder

½ teaspoon fine sea salt

2 cups (450 g) Cream Cheese Frosting (page 240)

1 cup (150 g) separated mandarin orange or clementine segments

1. Preheat the oven to 325°F (165°C) convection. Line an 11-inch (30.5 cm) round springform pan with a parchment round, coated with nonstick spray or brushed with softened butter.

2. Combine the butter, granulated and brown sugars, ginger, cinnamon, and orange zest in a stand mixer fitted with the paddle attachment. Paddle on high speed for 8 minutes, then scrape down.

3. Add the eggs, one at a time, and whip to combine well. Add the ½ cup (60 g) of chopped hazelnuts, the grated vegetables, and the pineapple and paddle to combine.

4. Sift the flour, baking soda, baking powder, and salt. Add to the butter mixture and paddle until just combined.

5. Place the cake batter in the pan and bake for 50 minutes until medium golden brown, turning halfway through that time. Remove from the oven and allow the cake to cool completely before unmolding.

6. Spread the Cream Cheese Frosting evenly over the single layer of cake, coating the sides. Top the cake simply with the crushed hazelnuts and the orange segments.

NOTES

To crush hazelnuts, place the whole toasted nuts on a cutting board and crush, using the bottom of a small, clean saucepan.

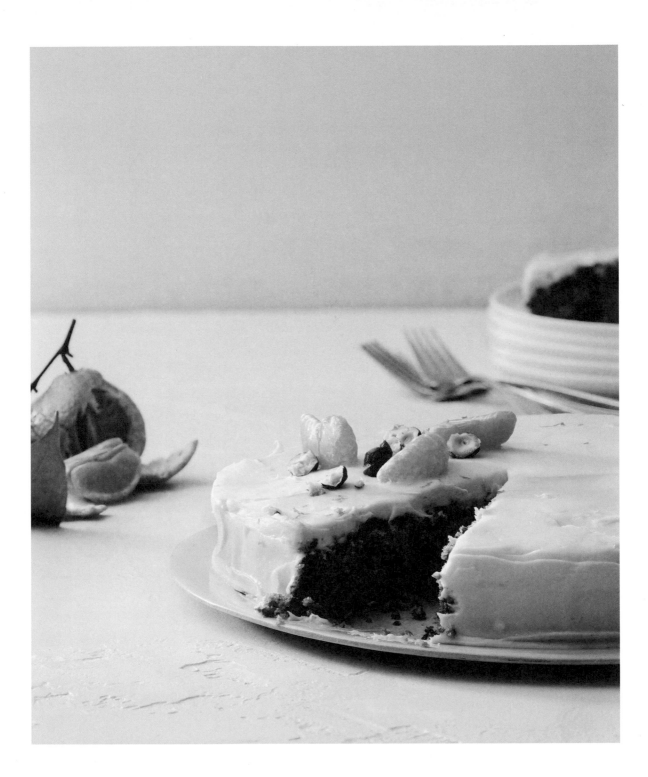

BURNT ITALIAN CHEESE TORTE

In the Loire Valley of France you can find burnt-to-black spherical cakes called *tourteau fromagé*. They are the strangest-looking things, but once you know what they are, they become a welcome sight. Blackened intentionally, this cake is a magical blend of goat, mascarpone, and ricotta cheeses, blended with rich butter and a small portion of flour. This is not even the same species as a classic New York cheesecake, but rather a creation all its own. The flavor of the delicious creamy cheeses shines through with the texture, which is a hybrid of a standard cake and a dense cheesecake. With a dollop of strawberry preserves, I find this cake to be utterly elegant.

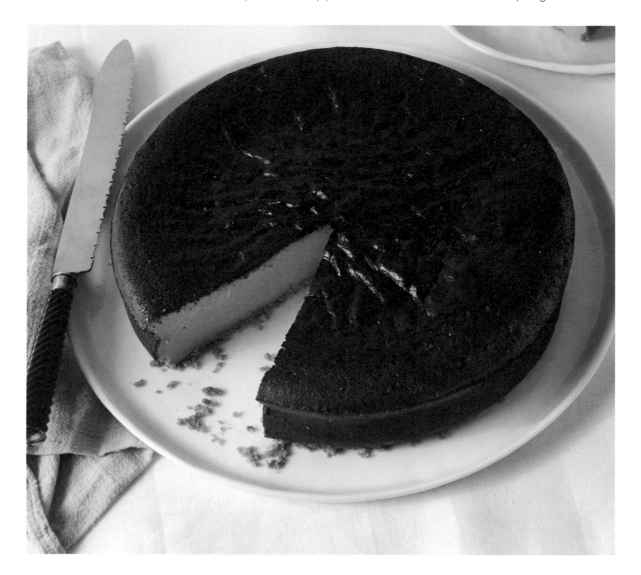

Makes 10 to 12 servings

SHORTBREAD CRUST

8 ounces (8 to 9 cookies/225 g) Classic Shortbread Cookies (page 142)

4 tablespoons (60 g) organic unsalted butter, melted

Pinch of fine sea salt

BATTER

8 large pasture-raised eggs (400 g)

¾ cup + 1 tablespoon (175 g) organic granulated cane sugar

¼ cup + 2 tablespoons (75 g) packed dark brown sugar

10½ ounces (300 g) mascarpone

10½ ounces (300 g) whole-milk ricotta

½ pound (2 sticks/225 g) organic unsalted butter, melted

¼ cup + 2 tablespoons (90 g) organic sweetened condensed milk

1 teaspoon pure vanilla extract

1⅓ cups (175 g) organic unbleached all-purpose flour

2 teaspoons baking soda

½ teaspoon fine sea salt

1. Preheat the oven to 325°F (165°C) convection.

2. To make the crust: Pulse the cookies into crumbs in a food processor. Add the melted butter and salt and pulse to combine.

3. Pack the crust into the bottom of an unlined 11-inch (30.5 cm) round springform pan, and bake for 15 minutes, or until just golden. Remove from the oven and allow to cool in the pan.

4. Meanwhile, prepare the batter: Combine the eggs and granulated and brown sugars in a stand mixer fitter with the whisk attachment. Mix on medium-high speed for 5 minutes.

5. Combine the mascarpone, ricotta, butter, condensed milk, and vanilla in a high-speed blender. Blend until smooth. Transfer the egg mixture to a large bowl and add the blended cheese.

6. Sift the flour, baking soda, and salt directly over the egg and cheese mixture. Using a large whisk or large spatula, fold the flour mixture together. This helps prevent the batter from splitting.

7. Pour the cake batter on top of the baked shortbread crust and place in the oven. Bake for 35 to 45 minutes, until baked through and golden.

8. Remove the cake from the oven and turn on the broiler.

9. Place the cake directly under the broiler to blacken for about 5 minutes. Do not walk away during this process! Turn the pan as the top blackens, to ensure an even burn.

10. Remove the cake from the oven and allow it to cool before serving. A dollop of strawberry or apricot preserves makes a lovely topper for this cake, or enjoy it as is.

NOTE

If for some reason your batter "splits" during mixing, where it looks broken or not a homogenous mixture, do not fret! Using an immersion stick blender, fully submerged, blend the mixture until it comes back together. This can be done directly in the bowl.

BANANA WHISKEY TORTE

Chocolate, chocolate, and more chocolate, bananas, Irish whiskey, and—you guessed it—more chocolate! This torte should be served in thin slivers, as it is so unbelievably rich and flavorful. There is just a touch of flour (but shhh, once to accommodate a gluten allergy, I had "forgotten" the flour, and it turned out just fine).

I made this torte when I was named a Top Ten Pastry Chef in America, opting for Japanese whiskey over Irish cream. Both work well, but the Irish cream is a bit less pungent than the Japanese, for a less booze-drenched situation. Winning that award was an unbelievable honor, as I represented the multitude of ways you could express being a pastry chef. I have continued the journey, showing that a good slice of chocolate torte goes hand and hand with a great yoga practice. Serve with a scoop of Clean Enough Banana Custard for a sublime combination.

Makes 12 servings

Nonstick spray or softened butter for pan

10 ounces (280 g) 70% dark chocolate wafers (Michel Cluizel preferred)

11 tablespoons (160 g) organic unsalted butter, softened

4 large pasture-raised eggs (200 g)

¾ cup + 1 tablespoon (160 g) packed light brown sugar

3 ounces (90 ml) Irish cream whiskey

2 tablespoons + 1 teaspoon organic unbleached all-purpose flour

2 tablespoons organic granulated cane sugar, plus more for sprinkling

⅛ teaspoon fine sea salt

1 large organic banana

1. Preheat the oven to 300°F (150°C) convection. Line an 11-inch (30.5 cm) round springform pan with a parchment round, coated with nonstick spray or brushed with softened butter.

2. Place the chocolate in a glass bowl in the microwave or in a bowl on top of a pot of simmering water, and melt until warm but not too hot. Gently whisk in the softened butter to emulsify.

3. Combine the eggs and brown sugar in a stand mixer fitted with the whisk attachment. Whisk on high speed for 6 minutes, until pale, ribboned, and voluminous. With the mixer running, stream in the chocolate mixture. Stream in the whiskey.

4. Sift together the flour, granulated sugar, and salt. Fold the sugar mixture into the chocolate mixture, using a large spatula. Pour the batter into the prepared springform pan.

5. Using a sharp knife, cut the banana lengthwise into about ten thin slices so that you have long strips of banana. Lay the banana slices on top of the torte to cover. Sprinkle the banana slices with additional granulated sugar.

6. Bake for 35 to 40 minutes, turning the pan halfway through that time to ensure even baking. As this torte is very dark, you will not be able to see browning; this torte needs simply to bake until the chocolate mixture is set.

7. Remove from the oven and allow the torte to cool completely before unmolding.

PIE!

I have had a hard time writing the word *pie* without an exclamation point for most of my life. Scrapbooking in my youth, I remember cutting out the word *pie!* from a magazine and feeling that I had captured my own essence for the mood board I was creating. I love to flex my creative muscle with pie, and this includes executing what I feel is my perfect version of apple pie, right alongside something new, including whipped yogurt, streaks of fruit, and a lot of dollops.

I am often inspired by other people when making pie. A custard tart may nod to the spices and floral essences found in Middle Eastern cuisine, or stir up a memory of family with the addition of herbs, which was ever present during my at-home exploratory process in the journey to becoming a pastry chef.

Pies can and should be made with different types of dough, in my opinion. Some pies, whether they are double crusted, single crusted, or blind baked and filled, call for a flaky, neutral-flavor crust. Other pies or tarts have a finer layer of filling and benefit from a crunchy, almost cookie-like crust. With less filling, which is often more pungent and creamy, a sweet crust seems to round out the flavor and textures more appropriately.

Pies are fantastic creatures, less precious than cake, but show your hand at creating dough with finesse: It must be sturdy enough to hold a filling, yet flaky or crunchy enough for textural bliss. Tarts are approachable and elegant, definitely something I always seem to end up sharing a slice of with a friend, two forks to a slice, whereas with the Doll's Coconut Cream Pie, do not even think of touching my slice. Taking care, getting to know my dough at all temperatures and consistencies, has been a great confidence builder for me in my pie making. The focus in the beginning should be on your dough. Make it nice or make it twice, as the fillings really are, in my opinion, easier to put together.

DO(UGH)

Hard-earned dough, produced with a delicate and deliberate hand. That is the kind that you can feel good about.

Truly great pie dough always starts the same way, with great butter and great flour and a cold, deliberate environment. Manipulating the Flaky Pie Do(ugh) to ensure pockets of fat are butted up against pockets of hydrated dough will in turn give you that flaky piecrust that we all crave. Doing a rough lamination, where you fold dough and butter layers on top of one another, further assists in that layered puff pastry feeling.

The Sweet Do(ugh) is beautiful and cookie-crunchy, a great contrast to creamy chocolate ganache, ricotta, or custard filings. This dough does not flake like its pie dough counterpart but rather crumbles, thanks to the granulated sugar and a bit of fresh lemon zest. Its density allows it to support richer fillings.

FLAKY PIE DO(UGH)

Makes enough dough for one 9- to 10-inch (23 to 25.5 cm) double-crusted pie

½ pound (2 sticks/225 g) organic unsalted butter, chilled and chopped into 1-inch (2.5 cm) chunks

2¼ cups (300 g) organic unbleached all-purpose flour, plus more for rolling

¼ cup (35 g) cornstarch

2 tablespoons organic granulated cane sugar

1½ teaspoons Maldon sea salt flakes

1 cup (200 g) ice cubes

1 teaspoon white vinegar

1. Place your stand mixer bowl and paddle attachment in the fridge to chill for 10 minutes. Place the chopped butter back in the fridge, in a separate bowl, to keep cold.

2. Remove the bowl and paddle from the fridge. Add the flour, cornstarch, sugar, and salt and paddle to combine, about 15 seconds.

3. Add the chilled butter to the flour and continue to paddle on low speed until the butter becomes the size of walnuts, about 2 minutes.

4. Pour about ½ cup (120 ml) water over the ice cubes to chill and then measure out ½ cup plus 1 tablespoon (135 ml) chilled water. Add the vinegar to the water and pour into the flour mixture in one shot.

5. Pulse the dough in the mixer by turning the mixer on and off, until it is very "shaggy," or a loose mixture.

6. Dump the mixture onto a large work surface lined with a large piece of parchment and gather, then pat the dough into a shaggy rectangle 7 x 13 inches (18 x 33 cm).

7. Using the parchment paper to assist, fold the dough in half lengthwise. Pat the dough into another shaggy rectangle. Using the parchment, fold the dough in half again lengthwise. Repeat this process four times more until the dough comes together.

8. Divide the dough in half into two rectangles, wrap with plastic wrap, and place in the fridge. Chill for 4 hours, to allow the flour to hydrate and the dough to rest.

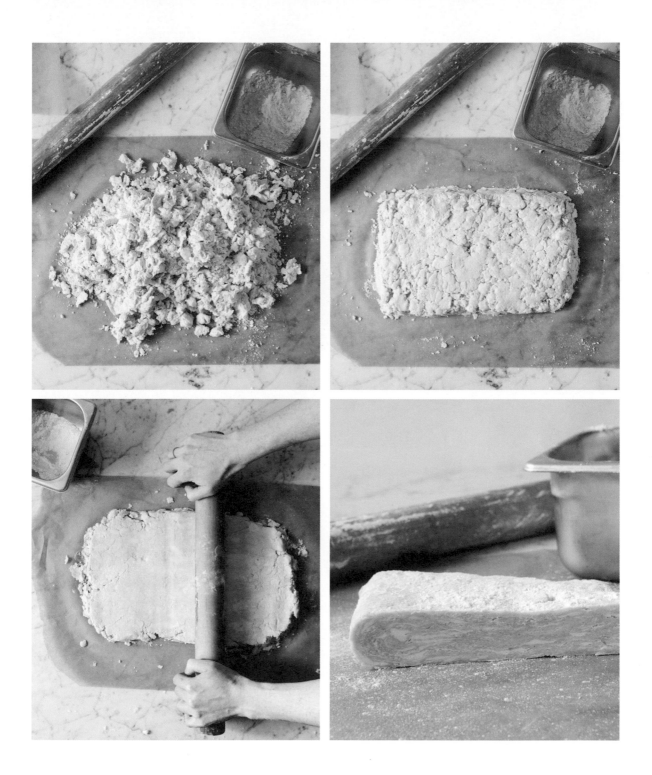

ROLLING DOUGH (FOR A DOUBLE-CRUSTED PIE)

1. Place a pile of flour on the corner of your rolling station—this is called "bench" flour.

2. Place the dough on a cool, parchment-lined counter or board and dust with bench flour.

3. Using the rolling pin, hit the dough a few times to soften it up.

4. Roll in a forward motion (away from your body), turning the dough and flipping it over as you create a circle.

5. Roll each dough pack into a large, thin circle of equal thickness, about 13 inches (33 cm) in diameter or large enough to hang over a 10-inch (25.5 cm) pie dish.

6. Place each circle of dough between pieces of parchment and store in the freezer until ready for use.

BLIND-BAKED PIE SHELL

1. Preheat the oven to 340°F (170°C) convection.

2. Remove one of your dough rounds from the freezer, leaving the second round for later use.

3. Allow the dough to soften up slightly, until it is pliable. Place the dough over your 10-inch (25.5 cm) pie dish and fit to line the dish.

4. Trim the edges to create a circle that hangs over the pie dish by 1 inch (2.5 cm).

5. Fold the exterior edges of the dough under to create a border, then either use a fork to press the dough down, or pinch between your thumb and forefinger to create a textured pie border.

6. Pierce the bottom of the dough a few times with a fork. This will allow steam to escape during the baking process.

7. Cut a large circle of parchment to place inside the pie shell. Fill the parchment fully with rice or beans. This will act as your blind pie filling.

8. Bake the pie shell for 30 minutes, or until just beginning to appear cooked instead of raw along the edges.

9. Carefully remove the weights and parchment, pat down any steam bubbles, and bake for an additional 15 minutes to fully cook the crust, this time without the blind filling.

10. Remove the pie shell from the oven and allow to cool completely before filling.

SWEET DO(UGH)

Makes enough for one 9- to 11-inch (23 to 25.5 cm) tart

11 tablespoons (160 g) organic unsalted butter, chilled and chopped into 1-inch (2.5 cm) chunks

1¾ cups (240 g) organic unbleached all-purpose flour

¼ cup + 4 teaspoons (70 g) organic granulated cane sugar

1 teaspoon lemon zest

1 large pasture-raised egg (50 g)

1 large pasture-raised egg yolk (20 g)

1. Place your stand mixer bowl and paddle attachment in the fridge to chill for 10 minutes. Place the chopped butter back in the fridge, in a separate bowl, to keep cold.

2. Remove the bowl and paddle from the fridge and attach to the mixer stand. Combine the flour, sugar, lemon zest, and chilled butter chunks in the bowl and paddle the mixture until it becomes crumbly. Add the egg and yolk and paddle until combined well.

3. Press the dough into a rectangle and wrap well with plastic wrap. Chill in the fridge for 4 hours.

4. Remove the dough from the fridge and place on a cool, parchment-lined rolling station with bench flour off to the side. Sprinkle the dough with flour on both sides. Using a rolling pin, hit the dough a few times to soften it (it will be very firm from chilling).

5. Using two sheets of parchment paper and bench flour, roll the dough into a large circle to about 13 inches (33 cm) in diameter, to fit the base and up the sides of a 10- or 11-inch (25.5 or 28 cm) or a 9-inch (23 cm) fluted tart pan.

6. Before placing the dough in the tart pan, chill the dough circle in the freezer to firm slightly, about 5 minutes.

7. Carefully place the dough in the fluted tart pan in one even sheet, pressing into the sides.

8. Place the dough back the freezer while the oven preheats to 325°F (165°C) convection, about 20 minutes.

9. Prick the bottom of the frozen shell with a fork and place in the oven to bake for 25 minutes, then turn the crust halfway around and bake for an additional 10 minutes, or until a light golden brown.

10. Allow the shell to cool before filling.

CARAMELIZED APPLE PIE

Growing up, I'd often find my Nannie near the bin in the kitchen, hand peeling apples with a small paring knife. We would have pie all the time and always with heavy cream poured straight from the pint on top of the slice. The cream was never whipped and there was never ice cream at the table. My Nannie's pies were different and I used to think that it was because it was the Canadian or more British way of making them: without cinnamon, sans ice cream, and always with vanilla. My Thanksgivings in the States, however, were where apple pie always had cinnamon, New England was bursting with apple orchards, and a tub of ice cream alongside apple desserts was ever present from September through the winter.

Now that I've taken pie into my own hands, I include both vanilla and cinnamon and appreciate a great glug of good cream before serving. The filling is also key: The best method involves precooking the apples so that the pie can be stuffed to the brim with flavor *before* baking, leaving no chance for fruit shrinkage. A variety of sweet and tart apples, browned butter, salt, and a touch of cream piled into flaky crust will make your holiday table swoon, no matter what side of the border.

Makes 6 to 8 servings

3½ pounds (1.6 kg/about 16) apples (Macoun, Empire, Granny Smith, Honeycrisp, Mutsu)

8 tablespoons (1 stick/113 g) organic unsalted butter

Scant ½ cup (100 g) + 1 teaspoon organic granulated cane sugar

½ teaspoon ground Ceylon cinnamon

½ vanilla bean, scraped, using both seeds and pod

½ cup (100 g) packed light brown sugar

¼ cup (60 ml) heavy cream

1 tablespoon fresh lemon juice

½ teaspoon Maldon sea salt flakes

1 teaspoon organic unbleached all-purpose flour

1 batch Flaky Pie Do(ugh) (page 158), rolled out and frozen

1 large pasture-raised egg (50 g)

1 large pasture-raised egg yolk (20 g)

1. Peel the apples and cut vertically into quarters. Cutting on an angle, remove the core and then cut the quarters in half lengthwise to make thin eighths.

2. Place the butter in a low, wide pot over low heat and allow it to melt and brown, about 5 minutes.

3. When the butter has browned, add the scant ½ cup (100 g) granulated sugar, the cinnamon, and the vanilla bean seeds and pod.

4. Add all the apples and then sprinkle the brown sugar on top of the apples. Sear the apples and then sauté to caramelize until softened, about 10 minutes.

5. Transfer the apples to a bowl to cool, reserving the cooking liquid in the pot.

6. Place the cooking liquid over high heat and whisk in the heavy cream, lemon juice, and salt. Bring to a boil.

7. Combine the flour and the remaining teaspoon of granulated sugar and whisk into the apple caramel. Boil for another minute, whisking.

8. Pour the liquid over the apples and allow to cool.

recipe continues . . .

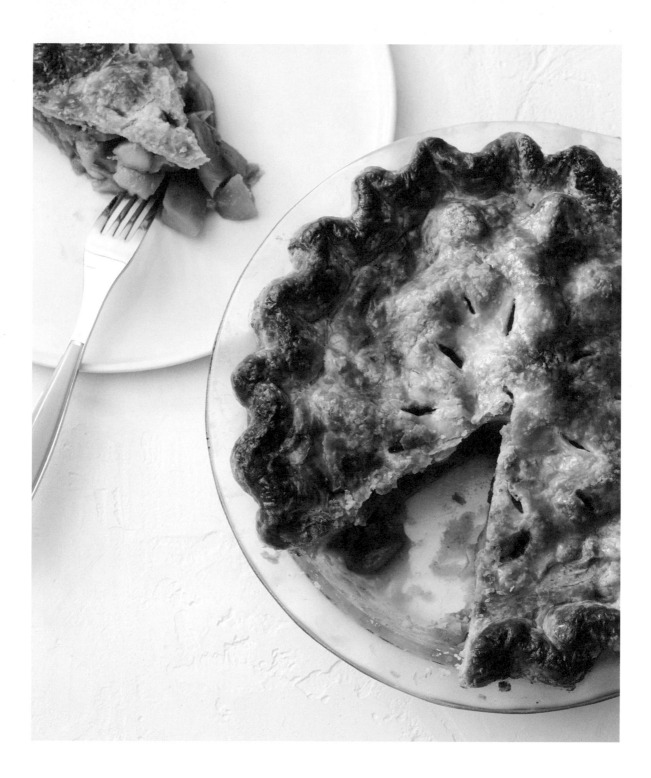

PIE!

9. To bake: Preheat the oven to 375°F (190°C) convection.

10. Remove both dough circles from the freezer. Place one dough circle into a 10-inch (25.5 cm) pie dish, with the edges hanging over. Pile the cooled apples into the dough-lined pie dish, being careful to not tear the bottom crust.

11. Place the second round of pie dough on top of the pile of apple filling, pressing the edges to seal both crusts together. Trim the sealed edges so that they are even, but still hanging over the pie dish by 1 to 1½ inches (2.5 to 4 cm). Fold the edge of the piecrust under and pinch the edges between your thumb and forefinger to create a fluted, sealed border.

12. Whisk together the egg and the egg yolk in a small bowl, creating an egg wash, and brush evenly over the entire piecrust. Cut slits in the center of the top crust to allow steam to escape.

13. Place the pie on a half sheet pan, which will catch any juices that bubble over. Bake for 55 to 75 minutes, turning halfway through that time, until the pie is evenly and completely golden.

SOFT CHOCOLATE TART

A tart is a filled crust, versus a torte, which is a single- or multilayered baked dessert that is more of a cake than a tart, but of a similar round shape. Tarts allow for simple ends to meals. They are great to place sliced on the table haphazardly with a pile of forks, encouraging sharing of a few sweet bites. While at the pastry helm of the Ace Hotel, I would make this dessert for diners coming in for large roast dinners served family style. After a very rich meal, a small sliver of dark chocolate was always the right answer. Serve the tart with a digestif on the side to bring your take on elegant restraint at a hearty meal's end all the way!

Makes 8 to 10 servings

Scant 1½ cups (360 ml) heavy cream

8 ounces (225 g) 64% percent dark chocolate wafers (Michel Cluizel preferred)

½ teaspoon Maldon sea salt flakes, plus more for sprinkling

2 tablespoons organic unsalted butter, softened

1 tablespoon Frangelico hazelnut liqueur

1 batch Sweet Do(ugh) (page 171), blind baked

1. Bring the heavy cream to a boil in a small saucepan.

2. Place the chocolate and salt in a medium glass bowl. Pour the heated cream over the chocolate. Place the butter on top of the mixture and allow it to sit for 2 to 3 minutes.

3. Using a spatula, stir the ganache together from the center outward for 2 minutes, until the ingredients are melted and combined.

4. Add the Frangelico to the ganache and, using an immersion blender that is completely submerged to avoid incorporating air bubbles, emulsify the mixture until the texture is homogenous, glossy, and smooth.

5. Tap the bowl of ganache on the counter to release any air bubbles and carefully pour into the Sweet Do(ugh) shell.

6. Allow the filled tart shell to sit, uncovered, to set in a cool but not ice-cold place for a day or at least 6 hours.

7. Once the tart is set, cut with a knife that has been placed in a jug of hot water, warming the metal, and then dried. Serve with a sprinkle of additional Maldon sea salt flakes.

NOTES

Instead of pouring the liquid ganache into the tart, you can pour the soft ganache into a container and store at room temperature or the fridge until you are ready to remelt it, pouring into the tart shell to set.

If your ganache cracks as the chocolate tightens over time, simply place the tart in a 275°F (140°C) oven for 5 minutes. The cracks will refill as the chocolate melts.

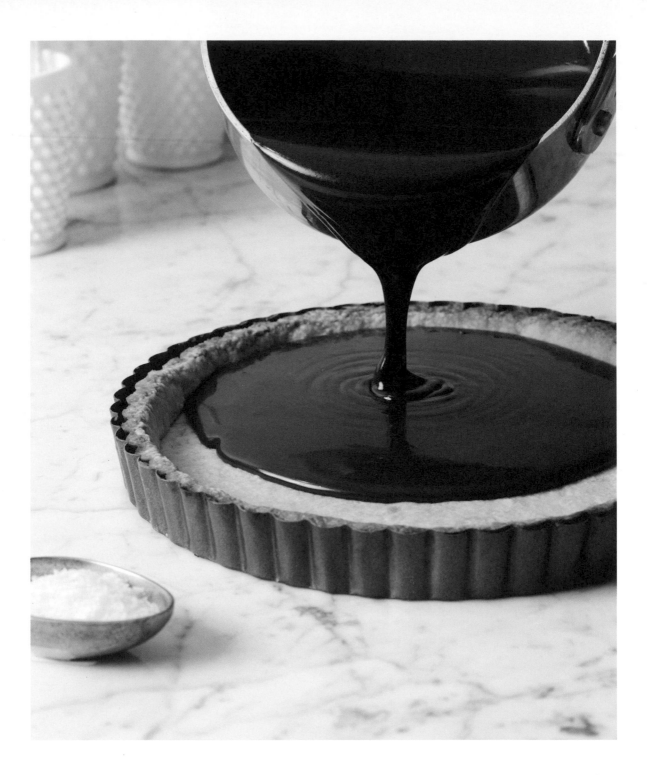

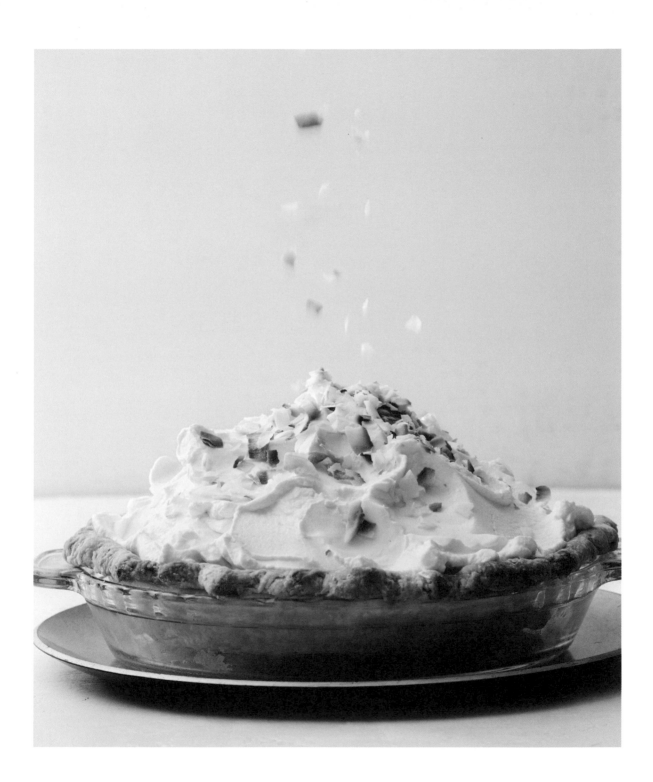

DOLL'S COCONUT CREAM PIE

My Nannie, Janette Dolina Guy, also known as the "Doll," was a tremendous baker. Did she cook? Certainly not. Grocery shop? No, dare I say never. Did she always have incredible homemade maple fudge, nanaimo bars, chocolate cake, apple pie, or coconut cream pie on hand? Absolutely. My Canadian side of my family loves sweets and is generally more of the British persuasion. All of us have a massive sweet tooth that can only be soothed by a proper slice of this pie. The Doll's pie has remained on the menu of my Uncle Robbie's restaurant, McKelvie's, since it opened its doors twenty-five years ago. They serve it as a colossal slice, piled high with whipped cream. I don't remember there being that much whipped cream on my Nannie's, but I bow down to the McKelvie's take on coconut cream, where it was served front and center during the celebration of her full and happy life. This pie is delicious and texturally balanced with a flaky crust, packed with coconut custard and desiccated coconut, piled high with whipped cream, and sprinkled with big toasted coconut flakes. You can't say no.

Makes 8 servings

1¼ cups (300 ml) whole milk

½ cup + 2 tablespoons (150 ml) full-fat organic coconut milk

½ cup + 1 tablespoon (120 g) organic granulated cane sugar

1 vanilla bean, seeds scraped and pod

4 large pasture-raised egg yolks (80 g)

¼ cup (35 g) organic unbleached all-purpose flour

1 tablespoon cornstarch

1 tablespoon unsalted organic butter

2 cups (150 g) unsweetened or lightly sweetened desiccated coconut

½ batch Flaky Pie Do(ugh) (page 168), blind-baked in a 10-inch (25.5 cm) pan

1. Combine the whole milk, coconut milk, 3 tablespoons of the sugar, and the vanilla bean in a medium saucepan and bring to a simmer over medium-high heat.

2. Place another 3 tablespoons of the sugar and the egg yolks in a bowl and whisk together to dissolve the sugar.

3. Stir together the flour, cornstarch, and the remaining 3 tablespoons of sugar in a separate bowl.

4. While whisking the egg yolks, gradually whisk in the flour mixture, ensuring there are no lumps. Then whisk ½ cup (120 ml) of the milk mixture into the egg yolk mixture. Transfer all the egg yolk mixture to the saucepan of coconut milk, still whisking. Place the custard on medium heat and whisk as it cooks for 2 to 3 minutes.

5. Whisk the butter into the finished custard, followed by the desiccated coconut, and transfer the custard to a glass bowl to cool for 30 minutes.

6. Transfer the filling into the blind-baked pie shell and chill for 1 to 4 hours in the refrigerator.

7. To make the topping: Whip the cream with the sugar and vanilla in a large bowl, using a large whisk, or place the ingredients in a stand mixer fitted with the whisk attachment and whip until the cream reaches stiff peaks.

recipe continues . . .

TOPPING

1½ cups (360 ml) heavy cream

2 tablespoons organic granulated cane sugar

1 teaspoon vanilla bean paste, or the seeds scraped from ½ vanilla bean pod

1 cup (75 g) unsweetened large flake coconut, toasted

8. Pile the whipped cream on top of the chilled pie filling and sprinkle generously with the toasted coconut flakes.

9. Keep the pie in the refrigerator until ready to serve. Use a clean and dry hot knife to cut into the layers of cream and custard when slicing.

VARIATION

For an even more intense coconut flavor, swap the ratio of coconut milk and milk inversely, using 1¼ cups (300 ml)coconut milk and ½ cup plus 2 tablespoons (150 ml) whole milk.

NOTES

If you end up with lumps in your coconut cream custard, simply strain the coconut custard before adding the desiccated coconut.

Be sure to continuously whisk the pastry cream once the flour is added, to avoid burning the bottom. You can also use a heatproof spatula to stir and get into the corners of the pan.

WIMBLEDON PIE

I have a penchant for having my interests become all-consuming, and my love of tennis is no exception. I love the sport, both playing and watching. I love the traditions, the casual sophistication, the sunshine, and in the case of the UK stop on the Grand Slam circuit, the strawberries and cream tradition of Wimbledon. Hence this pie, a hybrid of my twin obsessions for racquets and whisks. Named after that glorious tournament and created when tasked to make a dessert for a radio show while the matches were in full swing ten years ago, this is a beautiful cream-filled pie with tart Labne, sweet white chocolate, streaks of strawberry preserves, and studded with fresh strawberries. A sprinkle of bright pistachios takes it over the top. Enjoy this on a summer afternoon, in your tennis whites or not.

Makes 8 servings

1½ cups (180 g) whole strawberries

Scant 2 ounces (50 g) white chocolate wafers (Michel Cluizel preferred)

1 cup (225 g) Labne (page 109), at room temperature

Scant 1 cup (240 ml) heavy cream

3 tablespoons confectioners' sugar, sifted, plus more for dusting

½ vanilla bean, seeds scraped from pod

⅛ teaspoon ground cardamom

¼ cup (70 g) Erma's Strawberry Preserves (page 244)

½ batch Flaky Pie Do(ugh) (page 168), blind-baked in a 10-inch (25.5 cm) pan

¼ cup (30 g) pistachios, chopped

1. Remove the tops from the fresh strawberries. Cut half of the berries into quarters lengthwise, and the remaining strawberries into round slices. Combine all the strawberries in one bowl.

2. Heat the white chocolate in the microwave or on top of a double boiler, until melted.

3. Stir a spoonful of the Labne into the white chocolate, being sure to not allow the chocolate to harden and seize. Then fold the remaining Labne into the white chocolate.

4. Combine the cream, confectioners' sugar, vanilla bean seeds, and cardamom in a stand mixer fitted with the whisk attachment. Whip on medium speed until stiff peaks are formed.

5. Remove a scoop of the cream mixture from the bowl and fold it into the Labne mixture to lighten it, using a large rubber spatula. Then carefully fold the remaining cream mixture into the Labne, combining the two mixtures well.

6. Spoon dollops of strawberry preserves on top of the cream filling and sprinkle half of the strawberries on top. Gently fold these ingredients together just enough to streak the cream with preserves and strawberries.

7. Pile the filling into the cooled tart shell. Top the pie with the remaining fresh strawberries and sprinkle with the pistachios.

8. Place the pie in the fridge to cool for 1 to 4 hours to set before serving, then finish the set tart with a generous dusting of confectioners' sugar.

9. Using a clean and dry hot knife, cut the pie into slices to serve.

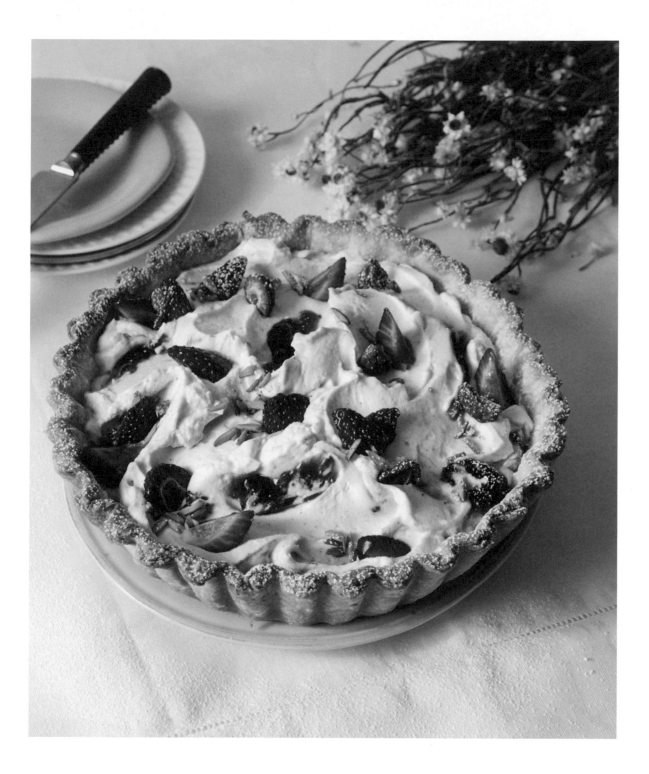

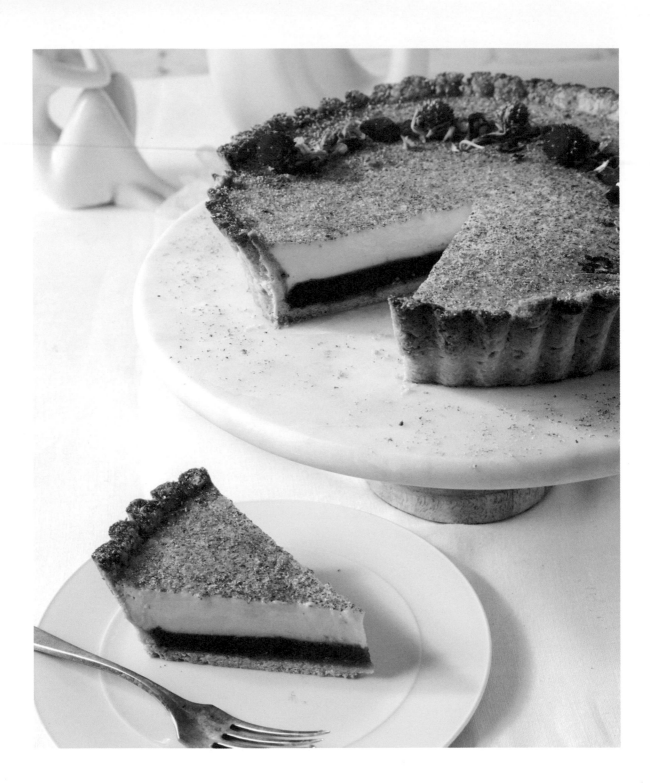

SILK ROAD CUSTARD TART

This British-inspired custard tart sings with the nuances of the country's imperial history: orange blossom and wild rose water pair with creamy custard bathed in nutmeg up against sticky sweet Medjool date puree, creating an international dance of flavor and texture. This is not crème brûlée and there is no vanilla bean to be found here. Vanilla, while a wonderful flavor, is not necessary for a good custard tart, whereas freshly grated nutmeg is essential.

Makes 8 servings

2 cups (350 g) juicy Medjool dates, with pits

¾ teaspoon orange blossom water

½ teaspoon grated orange zest

2½ cups + 2 tablespoons (660 ml/675 g) heavy cream

½ cup (105 g) organic granulated cane sugar

12 or 13 large pasture-raised egg yolks (240 g)

1¼ teaspoons rose water (Mymouné preferred)

1 batch Sweet Do(ugh) (page 171), blind-baked

1 whole nutmeg

Rose petals, dried rosebuds, and dried rose petal powder, optional

1. Place the dates in a heatproof bowl and cover with boiling water to loosen the skin. Let sit for 2 minutes, then drain the dates and peel away the hard outer skin. Discard the skin and remove the pits from the dates. Measure out 1½ cups (325 g) pitted and skinned dates.

2. Place the dates in a high-powered blender with 1¼ cups (300 ml) water and the orange blossom water and orange zest. Blend until smooth, then set aside to cool.

3. Preheat the oven to 290°F (145°C) convection with a low fan.

4. Combine the cream and sugar in a heavy-bottomed saucepan and heat over medium until just simmering or scalding.

5. Place the egg yolks in a bowl and whisk to just break apart the yolk structure without aerating. Temper the yolks, preventing them from scrambling, by slowly whisking a cup of the hot cream mixture into the yolks. Then whisk in the remaining hot cream mixture and the rose water.

6. Spread an even layer of the date puree on the bottom of the tart shell and allow to cool in the fridge slightly for 5 minutes.

7. Place the tart shell on a half sheet pan near the oven (less room for spills). Then carefully pour the custard gently over the date puree so as to not disturb the bottom layer.

8. Using a Microplane or nutmeg grater, grate a heavy coating of fresh nutmeg on top of the tart.

9. Carefully place the custard tart in the oven to bake for 30 to 45 minutes, until the custard is set and no longer jiggles when the pan is nudged, but remains soft without any cracks from overcooking.

recipe continues . . .

10. Remove from the oven and allow the tart to cool for 40 minutes at room temperature, then transfer to the fridge to cool for 2 hours.

11. Decorate the top of the tart with rose petals, dried rosebuds, and dried rose petal powder.

12. Keep the tart stored in the fridge and serve the dessert at a moderate temperature (between cool and room temperature rather than cold or warm).

NOTES

You can make the date puree ahead of time and store it in the fridge.

When baking a custard, you are allowing the protein in the eggs and cream to set, firming the custard, so the longer you cook it, the firmer the protein. If your custard breaks, you have made the protein too firm, not allowing it to carefully suspend the creamy liquid.

This dessert is delicious with Elderflower Cream (page 245).

JIMMY'S CROSTATA

Crostata, a free-form tart, is free from rules and loves life. I made this beautiful tart for Jimmy, who received this recipe in a very detailed format before I was even twenty years old. Jimmy is the only reason why this perfect-from-the-start crostata is even documented. His spirit is embodied in this perfectly imperfect creation.

Makes 8 servings

GRANOLA TOPPING

5 tablespoons (70 g) organic unsalted butter

¼ cup + 2 tablespoons (45 g) rolled oats

¼ cup + 2 teaspoons (40 g) organic unbleached all-purpose flour

¼ cup (50 g) packed light brown sugar

¼ teaspoon Maldon sea salt flakes

⅛ teaspoon ground Ceylon cinnamon

FILLING

23 ounces (650 g) ripe Comice pears, nectarines, or another sturdy, stone fruit (about 5 fruit)

1 teaspoon fresh thyme leaves

½ teaspoon fresh orange zest

½ batch Flaky Pie Do(ugh) (page 168), rolled out and frozen

EGG WASH

1 large pasture-raised egg (50 g)

1 large pasture-raised egg yolk (20 g)

Confectioners' sugar, for dusting

1. To make the granola topping: Combine the topping ingredients in a small bowl. Using your thumb and forefinger, pinch the ingredients together to form a crumble. Place in the fridge until ready to use.

2. To make the filling: Peel the pears and slice vertically into eighths. Place in a bowl and toss with the thyme leaves and orange zest. Set aside.

3. Place the pie dough round on a sheet pan lined with parchment paper and allow it to thaw slightly until pliable.

4. Pile the fruit into the center of the tart, leaving a 1½-inch (4 cm) border all around. Sprinkle the granola crumble generously over the top of the fruit.

5. To make the egg wash: Whisk the egg and yolk together in a small bowl. Brush the border with the egg wash.

6. Fold the dough inward over the fruit, overlapping, to enclose the fruit with a frame of pie dough. Brush the folded-over edge of dough with egg wash and place the crostata in the freezer to chill briefly, about 10 minutes.

7. Place the crostata in the oven and bake for 40 minutes, turning halfway through that time, until golden. Serve with a dusting of confectioners' sugar.

VARIATIONS

Fruit with a ripe, soft bite works best. I avoid berries, as they produce a lot of liquid.

If using nectarines, leave the skin on but follow the recipe as is.

The dish can be made more savory by dolloping some goat cheese over the fruit before topping with the crumble.

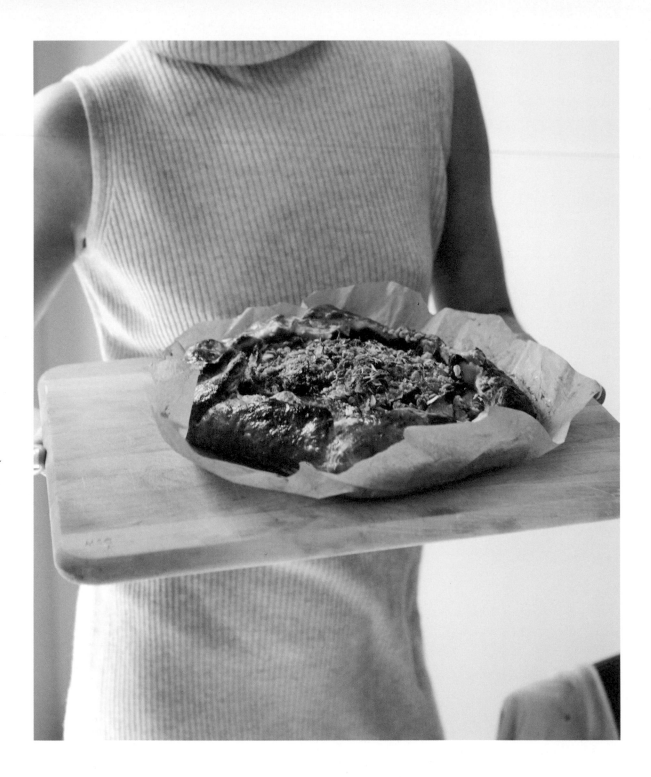

A LONG WEEKEND

Leisurely and long breakfasts—or their hybrid counterpart, brunch—are what great weekends are often made of. These breakfast-centric recipes are not for utilitarian weekends where the to-do list has reached a tipping point: Seductive Toast and blini stuffed to the brim with whipped ricotta are for the days that the bathrobe stays on. Beatrix Hot Cross Buns are planned for and baked fresh, feeding a group gathered with a similar weekend mind-set. These sweet muffins, scones, and morning buns pair well with the savory breakfast dishes, such as the Green Fava Baked Eggs or Israeli Breakfast and Soft Scrambled Eggs with Radishes, making a leisurely weekend spread truly Clean Enough.

As you read through the bread recipes, choose which one excites you the most first. The versatility of fresh brioche is a great place to start, leaving you with a loaf of enriched bread that can be made into various sweet recipes, the base for French toast, a delicious breakfast sandwich, or simply as is, possibly with a touch of preserves. Again, these are for the dog days of slow living at its finest.

After the sun goes down, dip into the luscious recipes for bites of versatile meringue, silky chocolate pudding, and creamy sweet risotto. They are great recipes to make generous servings of, feeding an intimate evening for four to a dinner celebration for twelve or more. Finally, plopping down a big bowl of mess—a mixture of fully dried meringue, fresh cream, and fruit—is and always will be one of my favorite ways to end a jovial dinner party. Messy and elegant, traits I absolutely admire in dessert and life.

CARAMELIZED BANANA MUFFINS

To a baker, overlooked and blackening bananas present themselves as a delightful opportunity rather than a waste of fruit. Save them! They make the most delicious banana bread or, better yet, Caramelized Banana Jelly, which is the secret to these muffins' rich banana flavor. Make a double batch of banana jelly to top a good bowl of Chocolate Puddin' (page 214), a more dessert-centric complement to these perfect morning muffins. Serve these warm with organic salted butter or Honey Butter (page 239).

Makes 18 muffins

CARAMELIZED BANANA JELLY

11½ ounces (325 g) ripe bananas (3 to 4), peeled

½ cup + 1½ tablespoons (125 g) organic granulated cane sugar

MUFFINS

Scant ¾ cup (140 g) packed light brown sugar

2 large pasture-raised eggs (100 g)

1 teaspoon fine sea salt

½ teaspoon ground Ceylon cinnamon

¼ teaspoon grated orange zest

10 tablespoons (140 g) organic unsalted butter, melted

1¼ cups (300 ml) buttermilk

½ teaspoon pure vanilla extract

2¼ cups (300 g) organic unbleached all-purpose flour

1½ teaspoons baking powder

1 teaspoon baking soda

1 cup (100 g) walnuts, toasted and chopped

Banana slices for topping

1. To make the Caramelized Banana Jelly: Place the bananas in a bowl and use a whisk or fork to mash. This puree will be fairly liquid if you use very ripe bananas, as you should, which have a high concentration of natural sugar.

2. Heat a medium saucepan over medium-high heat. Slowly pour in the sugar, allowing it to melt with each addition. Heat until all the sugar is melted. It will bubble and caramelize to a medium amber color.

3. Immediately add the banana mash, whisking to create a jelly. Whisk to break up any caramel chunks and then return the mixture to the banana bowl to cool.

4. To make the muffins: Preheat the oven to 325°F (165°C) convection.

5. Combine the brown sugar, eggs, salt, cinnamon, and orange zest in a stand mixer fitted with the whisk attachment. Whisk on high speed for 3 minutes.

6. Stream the melted butter slowly into the whipping eggs to incorporate.

7. In a separate bowl, combine the buttermilk with the vanilla. Reduce the mixer speed to medium and slowly stream in the buttermilk mixture.

8. Add the Caramelized Banana Jelly while the mixer is still running.

9. Sift the flour together with the baking powder and baking soda and fold into the batter, using a large whisk.

recipe continues . . .

10. Fold in the chopped walnuts, being sure to not overfold the batter, which will result in a tough muffin.

11. Line a standard muffin pan with paper liners and fill each muffin cup with a heaping ¼ cup (65 g) of muffin batter. Top with additional fresh banana slices, if desired.

12. Bake for 25 minutes, turning halfway through that time to ensure even baking.

13. Remove from the oven and allow the muffins to cool.

NOTES

Splitting these muffins in half and toasting in a toaster oven or underneath the broiler is the ultimate treat when they are slathered with butter or Honey Butter.

Make a double batch of Caramelized Banana Jelly and freeze half for future muffin recipes or to have on hand as an ice cream or Chocolate Puddin' (page 214) topper.

LOADED FRUIT MUFFINS

Eat with your eyes. This is a versatile muffin to fill and pile high with your favorite fruit. Whether bursting with blueberries, raspberries, figs or plums, the compote topping is just as important as the fruit inside.

Makes 18 muffins

FRUIT COMPOTE

11½ ounces (325 g) ripe plums or other stone fruits and berries

½ cup + 1 tablespoon (125 g) packed light brown sugar

½ teaspoon grated lime zest

1 teaspoon fresh lime juice

MUFFINS

3 large pasture-raised eggs (150 g)

1 cup + 1 tablespoon (225 g) organic granulated cane sugar

10 tablespoons (150 g) organic unsalted butter, melted

Scant 1 cup (220 ml/225 g) buttermilk

2 teaspoons pure vanilla extract

2¼ cups (300 g) + 2 tablespoons organic unbleached all-purpose flour

1 tablespoon baking powder

1 teaspoon baking soda

½ teaspoon salt

2 cups (300 g) fresh organic blueberries

1. To make the compote: Slice the plums, discarding the stones, and place in a medium saucepan along with the brown sugar and lime zest.

2. Cook over medium heat until the plums soften and begin to stew in the liquid that they release. Continue to cook for 5 to 10 minutes, until you have hearty plum compote with full pieces of plum along with cooked-down plum fruit. Remove from the heat, squeeze in the lime juice, and allow to cool.

3. To make the muffins: Preheat the oven to 325°F (165°C) convection.

4. Combine the eggs and granulated sugar in a stand mixer fitted with the whisk attachment and whip on high speed for 4 minutes. With the mixer running on medium speed, stream in the melted butter until fully incorporated. Slowly stream in the buttermilk and vanilla.

5. Sift the 2¼ cups (300 g) flour with the baking powder, baking soda, and salt. Gently fold the flour mixture into the egg mixture, using a large whisk, until just undercombined. Do not overfold; a few little lumps, as in pancake batter, are acceptable.

6. In a separate bowl, toss the blueberries with the remaining 2 tablespoons flour to help prevent the berries from sinking to the bottom and fold into the batter.

7. Line a standard muffin pan with paper liners and fill with a heaping ¼ cup (65 g) of batter. Using a soupspoon, create a divot in the top of each muffin and place a tablespoon of compote inside.

8. Bake the muffins for 18 to 20 minutes, turning halfway through that time, until they are a light golden brown. Remove from the oven and allow the muffins to cool slightly. Spoon an additional tablespoon of compote on top of each muffin before serving.

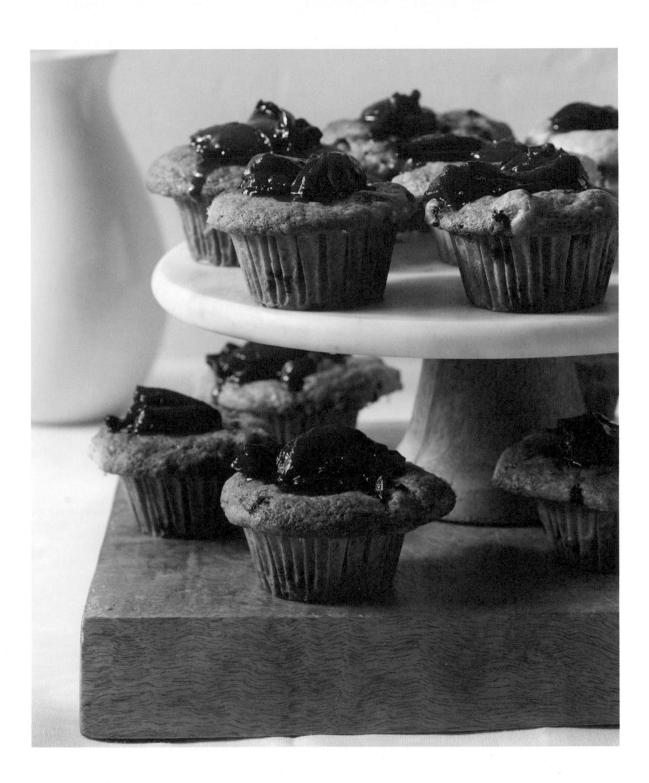

GROWN SCONES

I love hearty, flaky scones. Your typical scoop-and-bake scones may be slightly less involved than these, but there is nothing better than layers of light buttery dough, studded with fruit if you please, and with a crusty sugar topping for an additional layer of delight. Such a fresh scone, slathered with clotted cream and preserves and served with a proper cup of Earl Grey tea, is known as a cream tea, which I was introduced to on the little island of Guernsey in the channel islands of the United Kingdom. Guernsey, a rocky and gray island known for its dairy cows and subsequent clotted cream and cheeses, is the epitome of the right environment to tuck into this style of afternoon tea.

Makes 12 scones

12 tablespoons (1½ sticks/170 g) organic unsalted butter, chilled

Scant 1⅔ cups (220 g) organic unbleached all-purpose flour

Scant ¾ cup (75 g) cake flour

Scant ¼ cup (50 g) organic granulated cane sugar

1 tablespoon baking powder

1¼ teaspoons fine sea salt

2 large pasture-raised eggs (100 g)

Scant ½ cup (115 ml/120 g) heavy cream

½ teaspoon pure vanilla extract

TOPPING

1 large pasture-raised egg (50 g)

1 large pasture-raised egg yolk (20 g)

Scant ½ cup (100 g) organic granulated cane sugar

1. Chop the chilled butter into 1-inch (2.5 cm) chunks and set aside in the fridge.

2. Place the flours, sugar, baking powder, and salt in a stand mixer fitted with the paddle attachment. Paddle on low speed to combine well.

3. Add the butter and paddle on low speed until the butter becomes walnut-size. Using your hands, pinch the butter and flour together to flatten the walnut-size chunks of butter.

4. Whisk together the eggs, cream, and vanilla in a separate bowl.

5. Add the egg mixture to the flour mixture in one shot and paddle the dough together on low speed until "shaggy" or very loose.

6. Empty the shaggy scone dough onto a cool work surface lined with a piece of parchment paper and pat it out into a square, using your hands. Using the parchment paper to aid, fold the loose dough in half and pat into a square. Repeat this folding and patting process three times to bring the dough together, while creating layers of scone dough and butter, which will result in a flaky texture of the final baked product.

7. On the fourth round of folding and patting, the dough should be shaped into its final thick square. Place in the freezer to chill for 30 minutes.

8. Cut the chilled dough into six equal squares, being sure to cut straight down and not dragging your knife through the dough, which would pinch the layers of the dough together instead of keeping them separate and flaky.

recipe continues . . .

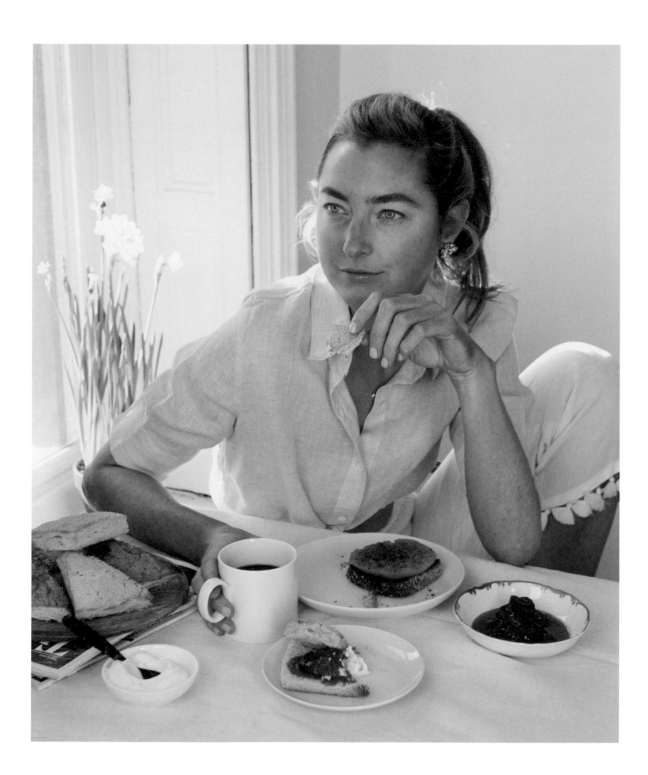

9. Cut each square in half diagonally, creating two triangles per square. Flip the scones over from how you cut them, so the bottoms are now facing up. This will ensure an even rise of the layered scone dough during baking.

10. Place the scones on a parchment-lined sheet pan and in the freezer to chill for 30 minutes to an hour.

11. Meanwhile, preheat your oven to 360°F (180°C) convection.

12. When the scones have chilled, remove from the freezer and make the topping: Whisk together the egg and egg yolk in a small bowl and brush the tops of the scones with the egg wash, being careful to not allow the egg wash to drip down the sides onto the parchment.

13. Using handfuls of sugar, heavily sprinkle the tops of the scones with sugar (1 to 2 tablespoons per scone), creating an even layer.

14. Bake the scones for 20 minutes, turning halfway through that time, until just golden.

15. Remove from the oven and serve warm.

VARIATIONS

Maple-Crusted Scones: Replace the granulated sugar topping with maple sugar.

Chocolate Chunk Scones: Sprinkle a heaping ½ cup (125 g) chopped chocolate into the dough as you create the rough laminated folds.

Blueberry Scones: Sprinkle a heaping ¾ cup (125 g) fresh blueberries into the dough as you create the rough laminated folds.

Cream Tea: Slather the scones with mascarpone and Erma's Strawberry Preserves (page 244). Serve with Earl Grey tea sweetened with a touch of honey and milk.

TAMARA'S BLINI

Beautiful St. Petersburg, Russia. A long walk past the Hermitage Museum, up multiple flights of stairs to an apartment that holds so much history. My dear friend Anna's grandmother Tamara lives in St. Petersburg and, despite our language barrier, showed me the kind of hospitality memories are made of one cold winter's day. The phone wouldn't stop ringing as the ever-popular Tamara seemed to be the epicenter of her social circle. Tamara made me fresh blini, slathered with honey and cream. As soon as I had one, another would appear. We ate and talked this way, swapping photos and laughter and pastries for hours. I was sent on my way back to Moscow with a large jug of homemade cherry cordial pulled from under the cupboard and a cheese and butter sandwich that I devoured on the train home. These blini, filled with whipped ricotta and folded into a beautiful flower shape, are drizzled with craveable Praline Honey. I know that they would make Tamara proud.

Makes 12 servings

BATTER

4 large pasture-raised eggs (200 g)

¼ cup (60 ml) brandy

8 tablespoons (1 stick/113 g) organic unsalted butter

Scant 1⅔ cups (390 ml/400 g) whole milk

4 or 5 large pasture-raised egg yolks (90 g)

1¾ cups + 1 tablespoon (250 g) organic unbleached all-purpose flour

¼ cup + 2 tablespoons (75 g) organic granulated cane sugar

1¼ teaspoons fine sea salt

Nonstick spray for pan

RICOTTA FILLING

7 ounces (210 g) whole-milk ricotta, strained using a cheesecloth, coffee filter, or fine-mesh strainer

2 tablespoons confectioners' sugar

Scant 1 cup (220 ml/225 g) heavy cream, whipped to stiff peaks

1. To make the batter: Whisk the whole eggs and brandy together in a mixing bowl.

2. Melt the butter in a small saucepan over medium heat and add the milk. Warm until the mixture reaches 120°F (50°C).

3. Whisk a small portion of the warm milk into the egg mixture. Then add the remaining milk, continuing to whisk. Whisk in the egg yolks.

4. Sift the flour with the granulated sugar and salt, then whisk the flour mixture into the egg mixture, being sure to break up any clumps.

5. Strain the mixture and store in an airtight container for 4 hours or overnight, allowing the flour to hydrate and the mixture to chill.

6. Heat a large nonstick skillet over medium heat. Then spray the pan with nonstick spray and remove the pan from the heat, ladling in 6 tablespoons (90 ml) of blini batter while swirling the pan, ensuring a thin coating on the bottom of the pan.

7. Place the pan back on the heat and cook for 2 minutes, flipping the blini over to brown on the other side for another minute.

8. Stack the blini on a plate and allow to cool before filling.

9. To make the filling: Place the ricotta in a bowl and break up any chunks with a large spatula. Fold in the sugar, stirring well to dissolve, then fold in whipped cream.

recipe continues . . .

PRALINE HONEY

⅔ cup (225 g) orange blossom honey

Heaping ⅓ cup (100 g) Praline Paste (page 233)

10. To make the Praline Honey: Combine the honey, Praline Paste, and ¼ cup (60 ml) water in a high-powered blender. Blend on high speed to combine.

11. To assemble: Spread the ricotta filling over half of each blini circle. Fold in half to encase the filling in a half-moon.

12. Fold each edge of the half-moon into the center, creating thirds. Fold this third triangle in half again widthwise, making an even thinner triangle. This will create a rose-like shape at end of the folded blini, where you will be able to see the ricotta stuffing.

13. Place the blini on a plate and drizzle with warm Praline Honey.

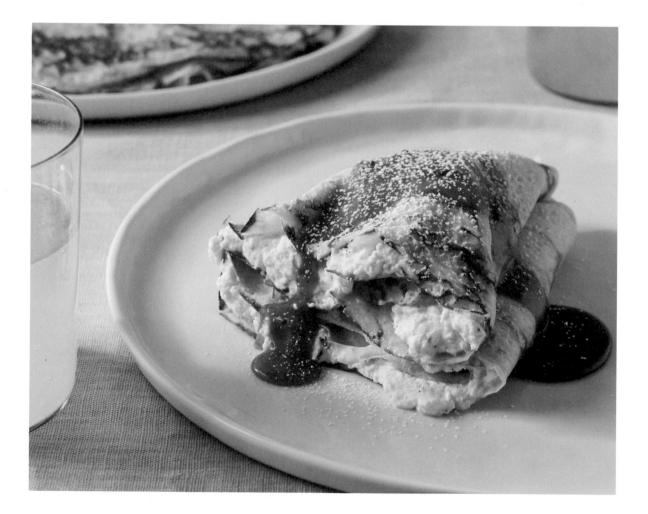

BEATRIX BREAD STARTER

A supersimple, keep-it-on-hand soured bread starter to make the breakfast breads full of flavor. This mixture is *alive* with natural yeast! I named my starter after Beatrix Potter, a favorite childhood author, but feel free to name yours as you wish!

Makes 1 pound (450 g)

Handful of Concord grapes, figs, or blackberries (½ cup/75 g)

1 cup (135 g) organic unbleached all-purpose flour, plus more for feeding starter

Pinch of instant yeast

1. Place the fruit in a cheesecloth or almond milk bag, allowing for easier removal.

2. Whisk together the flour, 2 cups (480 ml) water, and the yeast in a bowl, then transfer the mixture to a container large enough to hold the fruit. Add the wrapped fruit.

3. Allow to sit on the counter for 3 days, lightly covered.

4. Add 2 tablespoons flour and stir. Leave on the counter overnight.

5. The following day, add 2 tablespoons flour and 2 tablespoons water.

6. Continue adding 1 tablespoon flour and 2 tablespoons water to the starter daily.

7. On the tenth day, remove the wrapped fruit and discard. Continue to feed the starter to develop it for an additional two days, twelve days total.

8. If not using immediately, store the starter at room temperature, covered, in a clean, sterile container. It will keep as long as you keep feeding it flour and water on a daily basis.

SWEET BRIOCHE SERIES

A rich bread loaf with multiple personalities: excellent for Seductive Toast, Praline Toast, Caramelized Brioche (page 200), and, well, life.

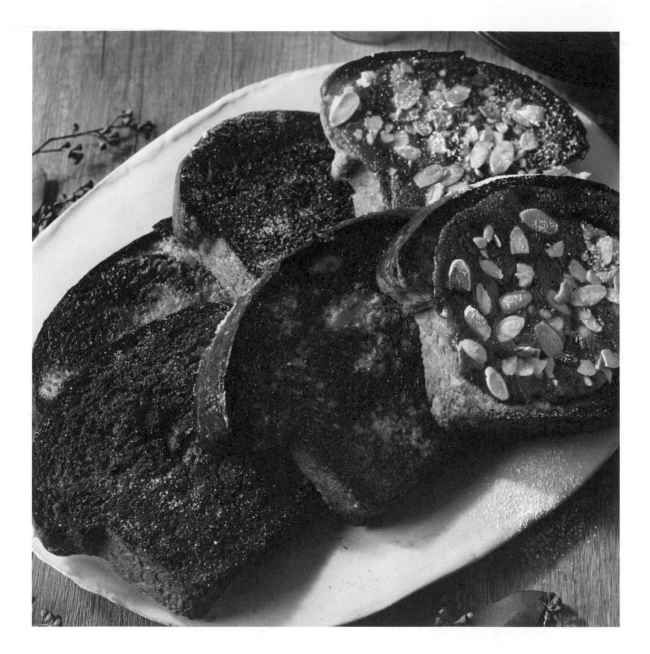

SWEET BRIOCHE

Makes 1 loaf

Scant ½ cup (55 g) plus 1 cup + 3 tablespoons (150 g) bread flour

¼ cup + 1 teaspoon (65 ml) whole milk

2 tablespoons Beatrix Bread Starter (page 197)

2 teaspoons instant yeast

1 cup + 2½ tablespoons (155 g) organic unbleached all-purpose flour, plus more for dusting

¼ cup + 4 teaspoons (70 g) organic granulated cane sugar

½ vanilla bean, seeds scraped

1½ teaspoons fine sea salt

4 large pasture-raised eggs, cold (200 g)

½ large pasture-raised egg yolk (10 g)

12 tablespoons (1½ sticks/170 g) organic unsalted butter, softened and pliable

Nonstick spray for pan

EGG WASH

1 large pasture-raised egg (50 g)

1 large pasture-raised egg yolk (20 g)

1. Combine a scant ½ cup (55 g) of the bread flour with the milk, bread starter, and yeast in the bowl of a stand mixer and stir together by hand with a spatula.

2. Top the yeast mixture with the remaining 1 cup plus 3 tablespoons (150 g) bread flour, the all-purpose flour, sugar, vanilla bean seeds, and salt. Allow the mixture to sit, unmixed, for 30 minutes.

3. Add 3 of the cold eggs and place the bowl on the standing mixer fitted with the dough hook attachment. Mix on low speed for 1 minute, then scrape down. Increase the speed to high and knead for 5 minutes to develop the gluten or protein structure in the dough. With the mixer running, add the remaining egg and the ½ egg yolk, scraping down. Add the butter 1 tablespoon at a time, allowing each portion to become incorporated before adding more. Place the dough, covered with a clean dish towel, in a warm place for 1 hour.

4. Punch down the dough to release the air bubbles and place in a clean, covered container in the fridge for 8 hours or overnight.

5. Spray an 8.5 x 4.5-inch (21.5 x 11.5 cm) loaf pan with nonstick spray.

6. Scrape out the dough onto a lightly floured work surface and pat into a rectangle. Roll out gently with a rolling pin to release any bubbles and fold tightly into a trifold, similar to folding a brochure. Place the dough, seam side down, with the top being the center of the trifold, into the prepared loaf pan, tucking the ends of the loaf under and creating a smooth surface. Allow the dough, covered lightly, to proof in a warm place for an hour and a half.

7. Preheat the oven to 385°F (195°C) convection.

8. To make the egg wash, whisk the egg and egg yolk together in a small bowl. Brush the loaf gently with the egg wash and bake in the oven for 15 minutes.

9. Lower the heat to 325°F (165°C) convection and continue to bake until deep golden, 20 to 30 minutes longer.

10. Allow the brioche to cool slightly before unmolding and placing on a wire rack to cool completely.

NOTES

Reserve the used vanilla bean pod and add to a container of organic granulated cane sugar to create vanilla sugar.

SEDUCTIVE TOAST

Scant ¾ cup (150 g) organic granulated cane sugar

2 tablespoons extra brut cocoa powder

2 tablespoons ground Ceylon cinnamon

1 Sweet Brioche loaf (page 199), sliced into six 1½-inch (4 cm) slices

6 tablespoons (90 g) organic unsalted butter, melted

1. Place the sugar, cocoa powder, and cinnamon in a dry blender. Blend to combine and slightly grind the sugar.

2. Brush each bread slice with melted butter and sprinkle generously with the cinnamon-cocoa sugar.

3. Toast in a toaster oven for 5 minutes to crisp.

PRALINE TOAST

1 cup (225 g) Praline Paste (page 233)

6 tablespoons (90 g) organic unsalted butter, softened

¼ cup (40 g) confectioners' sugar, plus more for dusting

1 large pasture-raised egg (50 g)

1 Sweet Brioche loaf (page 199), sliced into six 1½-inch (4 cm) slices

1 tablespoon crushed coffee beans

½ cup (50 g) sliced almonds

1. Place the Praline Paste with the butter, confectioners' sugar, and egg in a food processor and process to combine.

2. Spread a thick layer of the praline mixture on each slice of brioche.

3. Sprinkle with the coffee and coat with sliced almonds.

4. Toast in a toaster oven until crispy and golden.

5. Dust generously with confectioners' sugar to serve.

CARAMELIZED BRIOCHE

1 pound (450 g) Original Custard base (page 217), melted

½ teaspoon grated orange zest

1 Sweet Brioche loaf (page 199), sliced into six 1½-inch (4 cm) slices

½ cup (105 g) organic granulated cane sugar

2 tablespoons organic unsalted butter

1. Combine the Original Custard base with the orange zest. Soak the brioche slices in the custard base and then place the slices on a wire rack, allowing the excess liquid to drip.

2. Generously sprinkle one side of the brioche slices with half of the sugar. Use your hand to pat in sugar to adhere.

3. Heat a teaspoon of the butter in a nonstick skillet over medium heat.

4. Place the one of the brioche slices, sugar side down, in the pan. Allow to caramelize for 3 minutes.

5. Sprinkle the uncoated side with some of the remaining sugar, patting down, then flip the toast over and caramelize on the second side for 3 minutes. Repeat to cook the other five soaked slices, adding the remaining butter as necessary. Serve warm.

BEATRIX HOT CROSS BUNS

These morning buns are usually reserved for Easter, although they are a favorite of mine to make any time of year at brunches that I deem to be memorable. The buns do take advanced prep time, so give yourself a few days' start to get your fruits gathered before you make the dough and bake. Guests enjoy them most when sliced in half, buttered, and toasted on a griddle. Add a sprinkle of flaky sea salt before serving, and be transported.

Makes 8 buns

SPONGE

¼ cup plus 3 tablespoons (100 ml) whole milk

3 tablespoons Beatrix Bread Starter (page 197)

2 tablespoons bread flour

2 tablespoons organic granulated cane sugar

1 tablespoon instant yeast

DOUGH

2 cups (250 g) bread flour

2 tablespoons (30 g) organic unsalted butter, softened

1 large pasture-raised egg (50 g)

1 teaspoon fine sea salt

½ teaspoon ground allspice

½ teaspoon ground Ceylon cinnamon

Nonstick spray

Oil for buns (optional)

1. To make the sponge: Whisk the sponge ingredients together and allow to sit at room temperature for 30 minutes.

2. To make the dough: Combine all the dough ingredients with the sponge mixture in a stand mixer fitted with the dough hook. Mix on medium speed until the dough just comes together. Scrape the bowl down. Increase the speed to high and knead the dough for 5 to 8 minutes to develop gluten. The dough may seem dry, but it is not!

3. Combine the raisins, currants, and orange peel in a bowl. Add the fruit mixture to the dough. Knead on high speed for 5 minutes, scraping down as necessary.

4. Allow the dough to rest at room temperature for 30 minutes.

5. Punch down the dough to remove excess air and place in an airtight container in the fridge (with room for the dough to grow) for 4 to 8 hours.

6. Remove the dough from the fridge and scrape onto a work surface.

7. Using a knife or dough cutter, separate the dough into eight 4-ounce (120 g) portions. Spray the counter with nonstick spray and roll each piece of dough in a circular motion to create a round bun, with a belly button on the bottom of the bun.

8. Place the rolled buns, belly button down, on a parchment-lined sheet pan and brush lightly with oil or spray with nonstick cooking spray. Cover lightly with a clean dishcloth and allow the buns to rise in a warm spot for 1½ to 2 hours.

9. Preheat the oven to 325°F (165°C) convection.

recipe continues ...

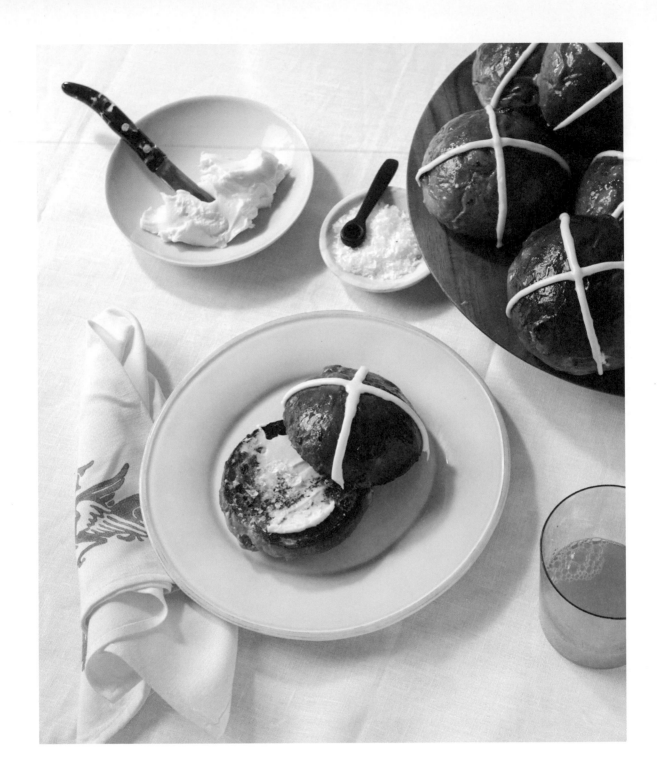

FRUIT

Heaping ½ cup (120 g) Earl Grey
   Raisins (page 243), squeezed of
   excess moisture

½ cup (100 g) Chamomile Raisins
   (page 243), squeezed of excess
   moisture

½ cup (100 g) dried currants

¼ cup (50 g) Candied Orange Peel
   (page 243), drained and diced, liquid
   reserved for glaze

EGG WASH AND GLAZE

2 large pasture-raised eggs (100 g)

½ cup (120 g) Candied Orange Peel
   liquid

¼ cup (30 g) confectioners' sugar

10. To make the egg wash: Separate one of the eggs, setting aside 2 teaspoons of the white to use for the glaze. Whisk the whole egg with the egg yolk in a small bowl. Brush the buns with the egg wash.

11. Bake the buns for 25 minutes, turning halfway through that time, until golden and even.

12. Remove the buns from the oven and immediately brush with the Candied Orange Peel liquid two times each. Allow the buns to cool.

13. To make the glaze: Stir together the confectioners' sugar with the reserved 2 teaspoons of egg white in a small bowl, then place the glaze in a small sandwich bag, cutting a tiny hole on the corner to create a mini piping bag. Draw a cross on each bun.

MISS MERINGUE

Making meringue is an incredibly versatile skill, and once you get the feel for it, the sky is the limit. Egg whites and sugar are really all that you need to know to be able to make such a wide variety of desserts; it should be its own book.

There are three basic varieties of meringue: Italian, French, and Swiss. They all achieve different volumes and have different methods of incorporating sugar into the foam structure of whipped egg whites. Without the yolk, egg whites contain no fat and are pure protein, which equates to strength—meaning, when the egg whites are whipped on their own without any added fat, they are able to foam and grow into a voluminous structure. The incorporation of sugar stabilizes the foam structure as well as adds a delicious sweetness we all know and love.

Meringue in and of itself is versatile and luscious, but when fully dried, it becomes hard as bones (as I like to say), adding a crunchy element to desserts. You can also can dry the outside of meringue, leaving a chewy marshmallow interior. When whipped, meringue is also a fantastic tool for adding volume to desserts, such as the Chocolate Stout Syllabub Mousse (page 212). Whipping meringue soothes any anxiety I may have, and piling mounds of finished meringue clouds on a platter or stand really makes me feel creative and accomplished, all made with a delicate and deliberate hand.

MERINGUE CHECKLIST

- Are your whites freshly separated? The fresher the whites, the stronger the protein structure. Why? They were just attached to the albumen and have not yet relaxed. Relaxed egg whites are better for the world of macaron.

- Are your whites room temperature? Room temperature whites will be easier to whip slowly and more consistently. They will accept the sugar into their structure much better than cold whites.

- Do you have a clean mixer, a clean whisk, and did you check to make sure no yolks made it into your whites? Fat is not your friend with meringue. Fat prevents the whites from being able to whip and make a bubble structure. Fat hides in unclean mixing bowls, whip attachments, and yolks.

- Break a yolk into your whites? Start over! Save the eggs for an omelet. Try working with a smaller bowl to separate the whites, frequently placing the whites into a larger vessel. This will save you if you break a yolk into the whites at the end of a dozen eggs. The acid (cream of tartar) helps break down the whites and stabilize the meringue. Cream of tartar is what turns baking soda into baking powder.

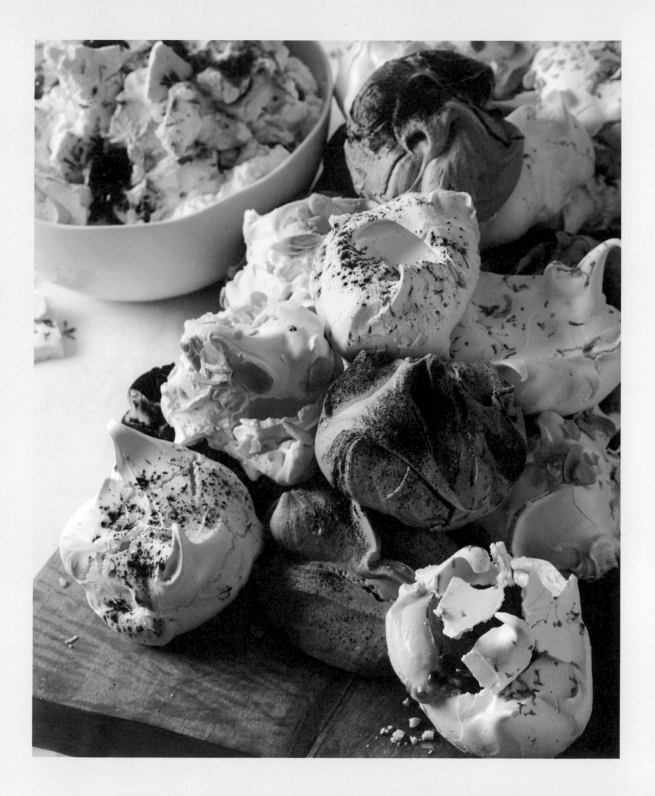

SWISS MERINGUE

Swiss meringue involves fresh egg whites, granulated sugar, and confectioners' sugar. Since you are warming sugar with the egg whites before whipping, you will be whipping a dense meringue. In its loosely whipped state, it is perfect for Biancas (page 145); in its medium state, it is perfect as a cake frosting; and in its fully whipped state, you can create beautiful clouds.

STAPLE SWISS MERINGUE

Makes 12 servings

7 large pasture-raised egg whites (200 g)

1⅓ cups + 1 tablespoon (300 g) organic granulated cane sugar

¾ cup plus 1 tablespoon (100 g) confectioners' sugar, sifted

1. Place a medium saucepan on the stove and fill with 2 inches (5 cm) of water. Bring the water to a boil and then keep at a high simmer.

2. Combine the egg whites and granulated sugar in a large glass or stainless-steel bowl and place atop the pot of the simmering water, creating a double boiler.

3. Whisk the mixture to warm and dissolve the sugar until the eggs reach 120°F (50°C).

4. Transfer the mixture to a clean stand mixer fitted with a clean whisk attachment and begin to whip on medium speed.

5. After about 4 minutes, increase the speed to medium-high. Continue to whip until the desired peaks or stiffness (loose, medium, firm) is reached.

6. Add the confectioners' sugar at the end and whip on medium speed to incorporate and then on high speed briefly to just combine. To use the meringue in Hot Mess (page 207) or Lime Clouds (page 208), continue running the mixer on the lowest speed.

HOT MESS

Makes 10 to 12 servings

1 batch Staple Swiss Meringue (page 206)

Zest of 1 lime, plus more for finishing

1 pint (300 g) blackberries, cut in half lengthwise

1 pint (330 g) raspberries

½ pint (170 g) strawberries, hulled and quartered

1 cup (225 g) Erma's Strawberry Preserves (page 244)

1 tablespoon organic granulated cane sugar, optional

3 batches Fresh Whipped Cream (page 245), whipped to stiff peaks

Confectioners' sugar for dusting

1. With the meringue in the mixer bowl running on the lowest speed, line two half sheet pans with parchment paper, using a dollop of meringue underneath each corner of the parchment to stick it to its pan.

2. Divide the meringue between both pans and spread out in an even layer, using an offset spatula. Zest the lime directly on top of the meringue layer.

3. Place in a 150°F (65°C) low- or no-convection oven overnight to dry out completely, anywhere from 4 to 8 hours. Do not increase the oven temperature or the meringue will brown.

4. Remove the meringue from the oven and store in an airtight container in large pieces until ready to prepare the Mess.

5. Place a metal bowl in the refrigerator to chill.

6. Place half of the blackberries and half of the raspberries in a separate large bowl. Using the back of a soupspoon, lightly smash the berries. If the berries are sour, use a tablespoon of sugar to release the juices and sweeten.

7. Add the strawberry preserves and mix to break up any whole strawberries. Gently fold in the remaining unmashed berries.

8. Using your hands, break the meringue into 2-inch (5 cm) pieces. The more haphazard looking, the better! Crush and reserve ½ cup (30 g) of the meringue pieces to use for topping.

9. Place the whipped cream in the chilled stainless-steel bowl. Add the broken meringue pieces and fold in, using a rubber spatula.

10. Spoon dollops of the berries on top of the cream mixture, folding in gently to create a very streaky mixture.

11. Carefully transfer the mixture to a glass serving bowl. Top with the reserved crushed meringue, lime zest, and the reserved raspberries.

12. Dust with confectioners' sugar before portioning with a large serving spoon into small bowls or coffee mugs.

LIME CLOUDS

Makes 12 clouds

1 batch Staple Swiss Meringue (page 206)

Zest of 1 lime

1 batch Creamy Lemon Curd (page 242)

Sorbet or ice cream of your choice (pages 220–225)

Fresh Whipped Cream or Mascarpone Cream (page 245)

Fresh cut fruit (try plums or berries)

1. With the meringue in the mixer running on the lowest speed, preheat the oven to 250°F (120°C) convection.

2. Add the lime zest to the meringue. (Lime zest has oil, so be careful to only add it at the end, as it can prevent the meringue from whipping.)

3. Line two half sheet pans with parchment paper, using a dollop of meringue underneath each corner of the parchment to stick it to its pan.

4. Using one large spoon, gather a dollop of meringue mixture from the bowl, about a scant cup (225 ml). Using another large spoon, scrape the dollop onto the parchment, creating a free-form cloud on one of the prepared pans. Repeat until you have a total of twelve clouds, spaced 2 inches (5 cm) apart, six per pan.

5. Bake the meringues for 30 minutes, then crack open the oven door (insert the slim handle of a wooden spoon to keep the door from shutting), lower the oven temperature to 225°F (100°C) and dry out the meringue for 30 to 45 minutes, until crispy, very white, and soft in the center.

6. Store the meringue in an airtight container at room temperature before filling. Alternatively, you can store the meringue in the freezer, resulting in the interior becoming chewy and the exterior remaining crunchy.

7. To fill, use your thumb to punch a hole in the bottom of each meringue or gently break the bottom off. Spoon in the lemon curd or use a piping bag to fill the meringue halfway. Then place a scoop of ice cream or sorbet inside the meringue.

8. To serve, place dollops of Fresh Whipped Cream or Mascarpone Cream on the bottom of a platter. Top with berries or cut fruit. Place the meringues on top of the fruit, with additional whipped cream on the side.

FRENCH MERINGUE

French meringue involves fresh egg whites, granulated sugar, and cream of tartar. The ratio of egg white to sugar is not as specific as in the Italian and Swiss varieties, which means you can adjust the sweetness easily to accommodate your add-ins.

Makes 10 servings

7 large pasture-raised egg whites (200 g), at room temperature

¾ cup + 2 tablespoons (200 g) organic granulated cane sugar

½ teaspoon cream of tartar

1. Place the egg whites in the bowl of a stand mixer fitted with the whisk attachment. Begin to whip on medium-low speed. The center of the meringue will look "snotty" as you begin to create bubbles of the meringue.

2. Once the thick whites are almost gone (i.e., foamy), add the cream of tartar.

3. As soon as the meringue has formed a full foam state, slowly sprinkle in 2 tablespoons of the granulated sugar. About 30 seconds later, sprinkle in another 2 tablespoons of granulated sugar. Continue this process, making sure to not add too much sugar at once. *You are building a meringue network here, which is a structure of tiny bubbles with sugar interspersed. This creates a strong meringue. If you whip too quickly, the bubbles will be much larger, which makes the structure weaker. If one big bubble pops, a great deal of the structure deflates. Small and mighty bubbles are the goal.* Patience is your friend during this process; it will only take about 10 minutes, but it may feel like longer.

4. Once all of the granulated sugar is added, add the confectioners' sugar while whipping on medium-high speed. This will make the meringue dense, which is needed for the Marvelous Clouds.

5. To reach stiff peaks, increase your speed to high for about 10 seconds. Then return the mixer to low speed for 1 minute to stabilize the meringue.

NOTE

Cream of tartar is an acid that helps stabilize French meringue.

MARVELOUS CLOUDS

Makes 20 clouds

1 batch French Meringue (page 209)

2 batches Fresh Whipped Cream
(page 245), whipped to very stiff
peaks

2 cups (250 g) dark chocolate
shavings

1. Preheat the oven to 250°F (120°C) convection with a low fan. Line two half sheet pans with parchment paper.

2. Transfer the French meringue to a piping bag fitted with a round tip ½ inch (13 mm) in diameter, then pipe circles 2 inches (5 cm) in diameter onto the prepared pans. Place the pans in the oven and allow the meringues to dry there for 1 hour.

3. Remove the meringues from the oven and allow them to cool to room temperature, then store in an airtight container until ready to assemble the clouds.

4. Place half of the dried meringue circles, bottom up, on a sheet pan. Using a piping bag fitted with a round tip ½ inch (13 mm) in diameter, pipe a double-tablespoon-size dollop of whipped cream on top of each meringue.

5. Place another meringue circle on top of the cream, pressing down slightly, to form a sandwich. Pipe an additional 2-tablespoon-size dollop of whipped cream on top of each meringue sandwich. Use a small spatula or spoon to coat the entire meringue sandwich with whipped cream.

6. Place the chocolate shavings on a small tray or a dinner plate for coating. Place the meringue sandwiches upside down (cream side down) on the chocolate shavings.

7. Rolling gently, continue to spread the cream and coat the entire meringue (except the bottom) with chocolate shavings.

8. Store the meringues in the refrigerator if you are going to consume them within a few days. Alternatively, you can store the Marvelous Clouds in the freezer up to for 2 weeks, thawing in the fridge before serving.

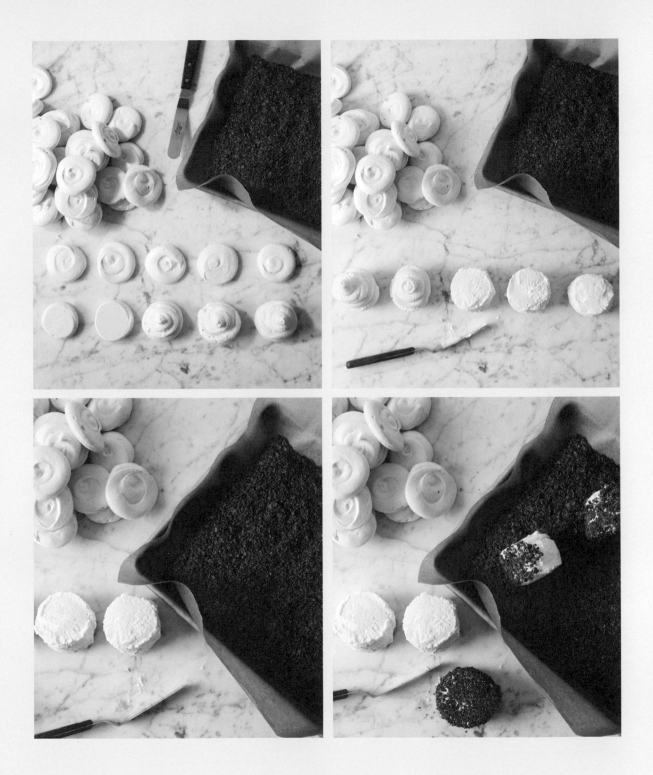

ITALIAN MERINGUE

Italian meringue involves fresh egg whites, a ball of soft sugar syrup, a touch of granulated cane sugar, and cream of tartar, all of which make it very stable. You can adjust the sweetness of an Italian meringue, but remember to use equal parts sugar to whites.

ITALIAN MERINGUE METHOD

Makes 10 servings

7 large pasture-raised egg whites (200 g), at room temperature

¾ cup + 2 tablespoons (200 g) organic granulated cane sugar

½ teaspoon cream of tartar

1. Place the egg whites in a clean stand mixer fitted with the whip attachment.

2. Place ¾ cup plus 1 tablespoon (180 g) of the sugar a small saucepan and add just enough water to create a wet sand texture. Using a wet paper towel, wipe the sides of the pot to ensure there are no sugar crystals clinging to it, which prevents crystallization.

3. Heat the sugar over medium-high heat. Once it comes to a boil, turn on the mixer and begin whipping the whites at medium speed. When the whites begin to foam, add the cream of tartar.

4. Add the remaining tablespoon of sugar to the whipping whites. This will help the whites accept more sugar when the syrup cooks. Meanwhile, continue to cook the sugar syrup so it forms a soft ball, about 235° to 240°F (113° to 116°C). Remove from the heat, add the bloomed gelatin if making Chocolate Stout Syllabub (see notes) and slowly stream the sugar down the side of the mixing bowl into the whipping whites.

5. Once all of the sugar is incorporated, continue to whip the meringue until it forms medium-stiff peaks. To use the meringue in the Chocolate Stout Syllabub Mousse, continue running the mixer on the lowest speed.

NOTES

Bloom gelatin by placing the sheets of gelatin in water until soft, squeezing excess moisture off before adding to the cooked sugar syrup.

The cooked sugar syrup, when placed in ice cold water, creates a soft ball. This is a precursor to soft crack, hard crack (such as a lollipop), and caramel. Soft ball sugar, when gently streamed into foamed egg whites, slightly cooks the whites while whipping, creating a stable foam structure.

If you overcook the sugar syrup, it will get caught in the whisk attachment and will solidify, without whipping into the whites and/or scrambling the whites from too-hot sugar!

CHOCOLATE STOUT
SYLLABUB MOUSSE

Makes 10 servings

4 ounces (120 ml) Taddy Porter ale or dark Guinness Extra Stout

4 ounces (115 g) 70% dark chocolate wafers (Michel Cluizel preferred)

½ teaspoon fine sea salt

½ cup + 1 tablespoon (135 ml) heavy cream

¼ cup + 1 teaspoon (65 ml) crème fraîche

1 batch Italian Meringue (page 212)

2 gelatin sheets

TO SERVE

Maldon sea salt flakes

1 whole nutmeg

1 batch Fresh Whipped Cream (page 245), whipped to stiff peaks

1 cup + 1 tablespoon (225 g) organic granulated cane sugar

1. Carefully warm the beer in a small saucepan over medium-low. Be careful not to boil, which will alter the flavor by destroying the alcohol.

2. Place the chocolate and salt in a high-powered blender and add the hot beer. Blend to emulsify.

3. Combine the cream and crème fraîche in a large, cold, clean bowl. Whip together by hand, using a balloon or large whisk, until very, very soft peaks form.

4. Using a large spatula, fold the warm beer mixture into the meringue, then fold in the cream mixture. Immediately pour the mousse into either individual 10-ounce (300 ml) drinking glasses or coupes or one shallow serving dish. Place in the fridge for 4 hours to chill.

5. To serve, sprinkle a small amount of sea salt and grate nutmeg directly on top of the mousse, then cover the top of the mousse with the whipped cream.

6. Heat a clean, dry sauté pan over medium-high heat, then sprinkle in some of the granulated sugar to melt. Continue to add the sugar in 2-tablespoon increments to melt before adding the next increment, until it eventually caramelizes to a medium amber color.

7. Drizzle the caramelized sugar directly on top of the whipped cream, using a small amount if pouring into individual portions. Swirl the glass to disperse the caramel and tap the glass down to allow the cream to bubble through the caramel as it sets. Top with additional grated nutmeg and serve immediately.

CHOCOLATE PUDDIN'

This pudding is everything you wish for in a more-ish lick-the-bowl-clean treat because it's essentially a blank canvas on which your sweet imagination can play. Simply serve it in glasses with a mountain of whipped cream and a pile of spoons on the table. Or let it be the base of dirt cake—which was the name of my first blog and the favorite dessert of my first love—made with crumbled Roasted Coconut Cookies (page 148) and Mascarpone Cream (page 245). You can also make it luscious with Caramelized Banana Jelly (page 188), fresh bananas, and Original Treacle Sauce (page 234).

Makes 8 servings

Scant 2 cups (435 ml/450 g) whole milk

Scant 1 cup (220 ml/225 g) heavy cream

6 large pasture-raised egg yolks (120 g)

Scant ¾ cup (140 g) organic granulated cane sugar

9 ounces (250 g) milk chocolate wafers (Michel Cluizel preferred)

4½ ounces (140 g) 60% bittersweet chocolate wafers (Michel Cluizel preferred)

½ teaspoon Maldon sea salt flakes

TO SERVE

1 cup (135 g) raw whole hazelnuts

1 orange

Maldon sea salt flakes

3 Roasted Coconut Cookies (page 148), crumbled

1 batch Mascarpone Cream (page 245)

1. Bring the milk and cream to a simmer in a medium saucepan over medium heat.

2. Place the egg yolks and sugar in a bowl and whisk until the sugar is dissolved and the yolks are pale.

3. Add a ladle of hot milk to the egg mixture, whisking to temper or warm the eggs without scrambling them. Then transfer the entire egg mixture into the pot of hot milk and whisk to combine.

4. Using a heatproof spatula, stir the stovetop custard until it reaches 180°F (82°C), or nappage, meaning the custard coats the back of a spoon.

5. Place all the chocolate wafers in a heatproof bowl and pour the custard over them. Allow to sit for 2 minutes, then add the salt.

6. Transfer the mixture to a narrow, tall container and emulsify, using an immersion blender. Be sure to keep the wand submerged, to prevent air bubbles from developing.

7. Pour the mixture into a shallow glass dish and cover with plastic wrap. Allow the puddin' to set in the fridge overnight, or at least 8 hours.

8. Serve individual portions using a heaping ½-cup (120 ml) measure, or simply make big scoops of all the set pudding into one large serving bowl. Store in the fridge until ready to add the toppings.

9. To serve, spread the hazelnuts in an even layer on a dry baking sheet and toast at 325°F (165°C) for 10 minutes. Remove the hazelnuts from the oven and, once cool enough to touch, rub the skin off. Grate the orange zest directly onto the warm hazelnuts and sprinkle with the salt. Chop roughly.

recipe continues . . .

10. Remove the puddin' from the fridge and crumble half of the Roasted Coconut Cookies on top. Top with an even layer of Mascarpone Cream, then sprinkle with the remaining crumbled cookies and the toasted hazelnuts.

11. Serve immediately or store in the fridge to hold for up to 6 hours.

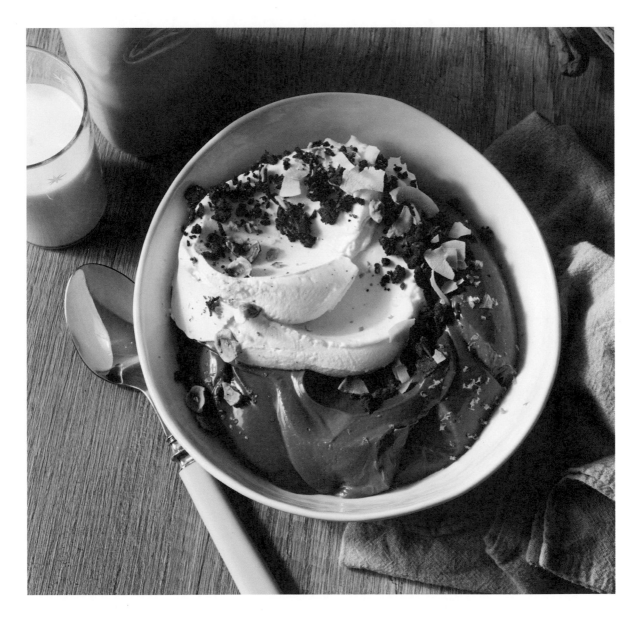

ICE CREAM AND CHILLY TREATS

Ice cream can and should be made at home. In this setting you have complete control over the ingredients, flavors, and fun. One of my favorite sundaes is simply excellent vanilla custard, swirled with my Original Treacle Sauce and topped with freshly grated nutmeg. A classic sundae that needs nothing else.

As we saw in the cookie section, ice cream sandwiches really take the cake for a post–rough day pick-me-up or a casual dessert. One of my favorite occasions for this was after a summer whites lobster dinner. The evening was a perfect mix of high- and lowbrow: lobster bibs, twinkle lights, and, of course, freshly baked chocolate chip cookies packed with Strawberry Shortcake Ice Cream. Fuel for a late-night dance party.

Ice cream also makes the ultimate milkshake. Do not skip over the Fudge Blitz or Halva Milkshake. They are sublime and appropriate for any occasion. All the milkshakes have ganache in them, so flip to the Sweet Pantry section to make M/D/W Ganache that is also a perfect sauce in a pinch.

Granita, both refreshing and creamy with espresso, will make a refreshing and textural end to a meal or afternoon siesta.

ORIGINAL CUSTARD

While working at the Ace Hotel, I used to make a sweet ice cream sundae called the Breslin Original. I would take big scoops of custard and hand fold in tasty bits *à la minute*. A little bit of brown butter curd, known as Original Sauce, is nothing short of magic, aged sherry jelly, caramel popcorn, and a bit of love. Every bowl that would come back to the kitchen would be licked clean. Not gelato, not American ice cream, this is *custard*. Frozen custard is rich, it's eggy, it coats your tongue in decadence. This batch is vanilla-free. Sometimes the aroma is a total crutch, as it's a standard addition to all things sweet. What about the taste of straight-up cream, milk, and rich egg yolk? Clean up your custard any way you can. When you have had Enough, serve with a swirl of Original Treacle Sauce and with a bit of freshly grated nutmeg on top.

Makes 12 servings

Scant 2 cups (440 ml/450 g) heavy cream

Scant 2 cups (440 ml/450 g) whole milk

½ cup (100 g) plus 3 tablespoons organic granulated cane sugar

1 whole vanilla bean, scraped seeds and pod

8 large pasture-raised egg yolks (150 g)

Pinch of Maldon sea salt flakes

1. Place the cream, milk, ½ cup (100 g) of the sugar, and the vanilla bean with seeds scraped in a medium, heavy-bottomed saucepan over medium-high heat. Bring to a scald (just before it boils). Turn off the heat and allow the vanilla to infuse the liquid for 1 hour.

2. Return the milk mixture to a scald. Meanwhile, place the egg yolks and remaining 3 tablespoons sugar in a bowl and whisk until the yolks are pale and the sugar is dissolved.

3. Ladle 1 cup (240 ml) of the hot milk into the yolk mixture, whisking, to temper the eggs without scrambling them. Carefully whisk the tempered egg mixture into the remaining hot milk.

4. Gently cook the ice cream over low heat, using a nonstick heatproof spatula to stir slowly in constant figure eights. This will ensure that you continuously scrape the entire bottom of the pot so that the egg yolks do not curdle. Cook the mixture to 180°F (82°C) and the custard coats the back of a spoon without dripping (see "nappage" on page 134), then immediately pour the mixture into a bowl set over a bowl of ice to cool rapidly.

5. Once your ice cream has reached room temperature in the ice bath, place the mixture in a container in the fridge overnight to allow the custard to settle and gel.

6. The next day, whisk the mixture and strain it through a fine-mesh strainer, using a ladle to push everything through.

7. Whisk in a pinch of salt and spin according to the manufacturer's directions for your ice cream machine.

8. Store in a container in the freezer to firm further.

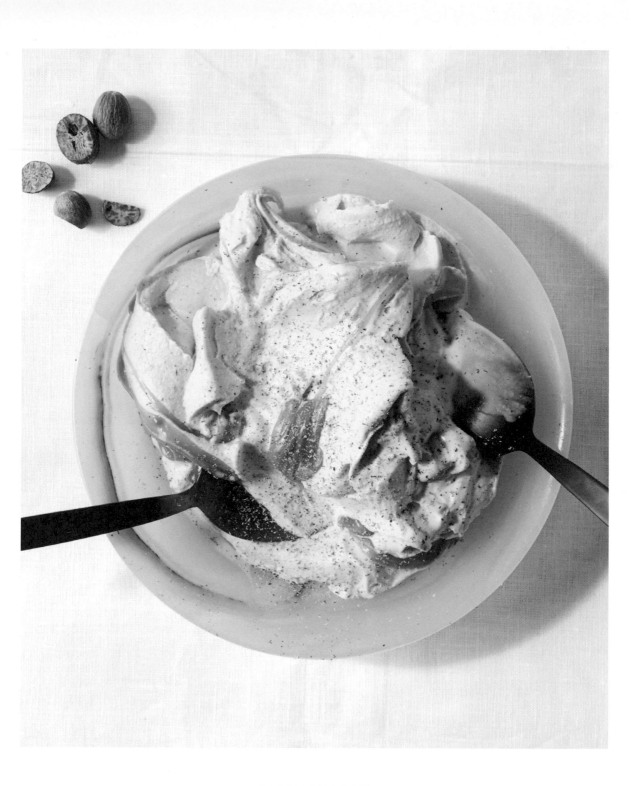

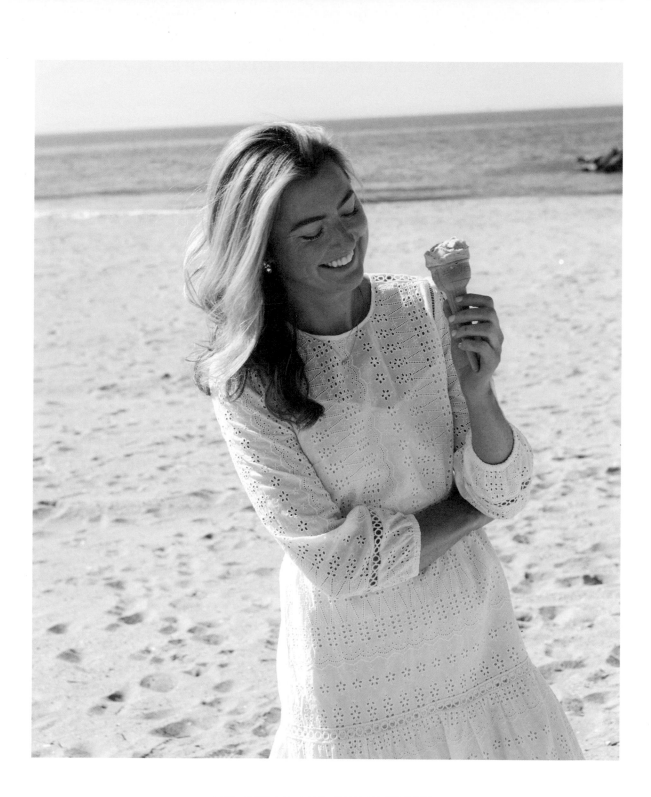

ICE CREAM AND CHILLY TREATS

JIM WELU'S CINNAMON ICE CREAM

As a child, I would mosey over to my neighbor Jim Welu's house weekly; I would arrive with my best friend, Caroline, for a visit, which would involve our selling him something like a glitterized rock, or singing him a song that I wrote. These weekly visits were always code for Cinnamon Ice Cream. Jim was the director of the Worcester Art Museum by day and an avid ice cream maker by night. To this day, I still eat his ice cream every Christmas when I go home for his annual party.

Makes 8 servings

Scant 1¼ cups (290 ml/300 g) heavy cream

Scant 1¼ cups (290 ml/300 g) whole milk

¼ cup plus 3 tablespoons (100 ml) pure maple syrup

1 tablespoon ground Ceylon cinnamon

5 large pasture-raised egg yolks (100 g)

½ cup + 1 tablespoon (115 g) organic granulated cane sugar

2 Ceylon cinnamon sticks

1. Preheat the oven to 350°F (180°C) convection.

2. Combine the cream, milk, maple syrup, and ground cinnamon in a medium, heavy-bottomed saucepan and place over medium heat to warm just before scalding.

3. Place the cinnamon sticks in the oven for 5 minutes to toast before adding to the warmed milk mixture. Remove the mixture from the heat and allow to sit for 1 hour at room temperature.

4. Return the milk to the stove and bring it to a scald (just before it boils). Meanwhile, place the egg yolks and sugar in a bowl and whisk until the yolks are pale and the sugar is dissolved.

5. Ladle 1 cup (240 ml) of the hot milk into the egg mixture while whisking. Carefully whisk the tempered egg mixture into the remaining hot milk. Remove the cinnamon sticks.

6. Cook the custard over medium-low heat, stirring constantly with a heatproof spatula, until it reaches 180°F (82°C) and the custard coats the back of a spoon without dripping.

7. Immediately remove the custard from the heat and strain through a fine-mesh strainer to catch any remaining egg particles.

8. Add the cinnamon sticks back to the custard and pour the mixture into a bowl set over a trough of ice to cool rapidly, stirring occasionally until it reaches room temperature.

9. Place the custard in an airtight container in the fridge overnight to cool and gel.

10. Spin the ice cream according to the manufacturer's directions for your ice cream machine. Store in a container in the freezer to firm further.

WHIPPED CREAM GLACÉ

If you have ever ventured to London in the summer, you may have come across Flake ice cream. This is a white ice cream–like mixture that has a Nestlé Flake candy bar stuck in the cone. Whipped Cream Glacé is also a great representation of the ice cream accompanying the Flake, but made with real organic whole milk and cream. Whipping the cream prior to whisking it into the base adds a lightness to the ice cream that is intentional. Serve this inside a rich Roasted Coconut Cookie (page 148) for a game of balance. It is as light, crisp, creamy, and refreshing as it is decadent.

Makes 8 servings

2 cups (480 ml/500 g) whole milk

¼ cup plus 3 tablespoons (100 g) organic corn syrup

1 teaspoon pure vanilla extract

¼ cup (20 g) powdered dry milk

2 tablespoons organic granulated cane sugar

Scant 2 cups (435 ml/450 g) heavy cream

1. Place the milk, corn syrup, and vanilla in a high-powered blender and blend to combine.

2. Combine the powdered milk with the sugar in a small bowl to disperse the powder and prevent clumping, then add to the blender. Blend on high speed for 1 minute.

3. Whip the cream in a stand mixer fitted with the whisk attachment until it reaches medium-soft peaks, about 3 minutes.

4. Fold together the milk mixture and cream by hand, with a whisk, and spin immediately according to the manufacturer's directions for your ice cream machine.

5. Store in an airtight container in the freezer.

STRAWBERRY SHORTCAKE ICE CREAM

When in dessert doubt, I encourage you to do this: Get the sweetest, most delicious strawberries you can find. Slice them into quarters into a small, dainty bowl. Pour a few tablespoons of the best-quality cream over the top and serve with a demitasse spoon or a petite fork. There really is something utterly magical about cream and strawberries, and this ice cream, while requiring a few more steps than cut and pour, feels equally sweet and simple.

Makes 12 servings

17½ ounces (about 3½ cups/500 g) fresh ripe strawberries, hulled

3 tablespoons organic corn syrup

3⅔ cups (880 ml/900 g) heavy cream

1 whole vanilla bean, scraped seeds and pod

9 large pasture-raised egg yolks (180 g)

Scant ¾ cup (150 g) organic granulated cane sugar

1 teaspoon fresh lemon juice

Pinch of Maldon sea salt flakes

1 teaspoon rose water (Mymouné preferred), optional

1. Combine 9½ ounces (scant 2 cups/275 g) of the strawberries with the corn syrup in a high-powered blender. Blend until smooth, then transfer the mixture to a medium, heavy-bottomed saucepan and heat to a simmer over medium heat, whisking for 3 minutes to cook slightly. Remove the puree from the heat and allow to cool in a separate container.

2. In the same medium pot, combine the cream and vanilla bean with ¼ cup (50 g) of the sugar. Bring to a scald (just before it boils).

3. Meanwhile, combine the egg yolks and the remaining sugar in a bowl and whisk until the yolks are pale and the sugar is dissolved.

4. Ladle 1 cup (240 ml) of the hot cream into the yolk mixture while whisking and then whisk the tempered egg mixture into the pot.

5. Cook the custard over medium heat, stirring constantly with a heatproof spatula, until it reaches 180°F (82°C) and the custard coats the back of a spoon without dripping.

6. Immediately remove the custard from the heat and strain through a fine-mesh strainer into a bowl set over a bowl of ice to cool.

7. Place the remaining whole strawberries, strawberry puree, lemon juice, and salt in a high-powdered blender and blend until there are still some chunks in the mixture. Whisk the strawberry mixture and rose water, if using, into the cooled custard and place in the fridge overnight.

8. Spin according to the manufacturer's directions for your ice cream machine and store in a container in the freezer to firm further.

NOTE

Serve this ice cream with the Classic Shortbread cookies (page 142) or a slice of Pan di Spagna (page 156) or Silk Road Custard Tart (page 183).

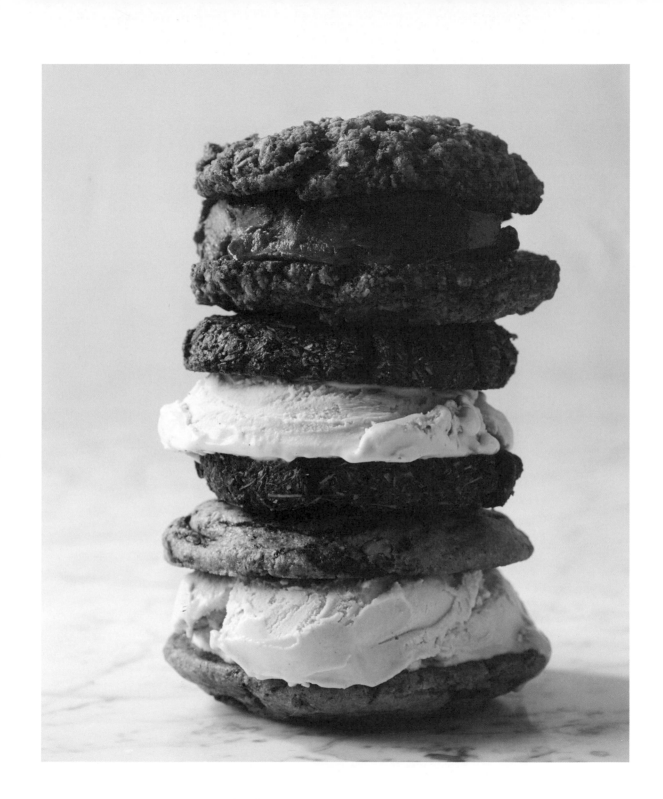

PISTACHIO PISTACHIO

Pistachio is a favorite flavor, color, and ingredient in my life: flavorful, vibrant, and a little luxurious. I prefer to make this gelato using whole pistachios, rather than store-bought pistachio paste. With the multitude of varieties of pistachios available, choose the one you like the best. I prefer using a combination of highly coveted Sicilian pistachios, which have an almost coconut-like aroma, along with hearty Californian pistachios.

Makes 8 servings

Scant 1½ cups (350 ml/360 g) heavy cream

¾ cup + 1½ tablespoons (205 ml/210 g) whole milk

¼ cup + 2 tablespoons (90 g) organic full-fat coconut milk

2⅓ cups (300 g) unsalted raw pistachios

¼ cup (50 g) organic granulated cane sugar

1 tablespoon cornstarch

¼ teaspoon Maldon sea salt flakes

1. Preheat the oven to 300°F (150°C) convection.

2. Combine the cream, milk, and coconut milk in a small, heavy-bottomed saucepan and heat over medium-high heat to a scald (just before it boils).

3. Meanwhile, place the pistachios in a single layer on a sheet pan. Toast for 5 minutes in the oven to just warm, not brown. (Do not overtoast them! You simply need to toast them slightly to heat the oils in the nuts and allow for better infusion.)

4. Reserving ⅓ cup (40 g) of the pistachios, add the remaining hot pistachios to the hot cream mixture.

5. Blend the mixture in a high-powdered blender on high speed for 3 minutes, then allow to cool and sit for 1 hour.

6. Return the mixture to a saucepan over medium heat. Meanwhile, whisk together the sugar and cornstarch in a small bowl, then whisk into the warming pistachio milk and cook for 2 minutes.

7. Strain the mixture, using a small ladle to press out all of the liquid.

8. Finely chop the reserved pistachios and whisk into the mixture along with the salt.

9. Cool the mixture in the fridge overnight.

10. Spin according to the manufacturer's directions for your ice cream machine and store in a container in the freezer to firm further.

RASPBERRY FIG SORBET

This sorbet base can be used for any fruit or fruit combination you wish. The key is to get a smooth puree, sweetened just enough to be a treat and prevent ice crystals when spinning in the ice cream machine. Among many other things, Sherry Yard taught me the secret to this sorbet: Add a bit of Pellegrino to the mixture to lighten it up and offer an elegant mineral undertone. That notion of adding touches of elegance to my desserts has stuck with me, sorbet being a refined moment in the course of a meal, after all.

Makes 6 servings

½ Ceylon cinnamon stick

8 ounces (225 g) fresh raspberries, pureed and strained

8 ounces (225 g) whole fresh figs, pureed in a high-powered blender and strained

¼ cup + 1 to 2 tablespoons (75 to 90 ml) organic corn syrup (see Notes)

1 tablespoon fresh lemon juice

¼ cup + 1 tablespoon (75 ml) Pellegrino

Pinch of salt

1. Preheat the oven to 325°F (165°C) convection. Toast the cinnamon stick in the oven until fragrant, about 5 minutes.

2. Blend the strained fruit puree with the corn syrup and lemon juice, using a whisk or high-powered blender.

3. Add the toasted cinnamon stick to infuse for 1 hour.

4. Remove the cinnamon and whisk in the Pellegrino and salt.

5. Spin according to the manufacturer's directions for your ice cream machine.

6. Store in a container in the freezer to firm further.

NOTE

Adjust the corn syrup based on the sweetness of the fruit. Figs are inherently very sweet, but if you are using only raspberries, you may add more syrup to taste.

CLEAN ENOUGH BANANA CUSTARD

Bananas offer so much to a variety of Clean Enough foods. This custard calls upon the flavor of a ripe, just-beginning-to-speckle banana. Some of the starchiness remains as it cooks and gets preserved when immediately strained. This ice cream on top of the Banana Whiskey Torte (page 166) may very well send you to heaven. But I dare you to be different and try a scoop inside Tea Raisin Oatmeal Cookies (page 139) for a combination you most likely have never tried.

Makes 10 servings

Scant 2 cups (440 ml/450 g) whole milk

3 ripe bananas, peeled

Three 2-inch (5 cm) strips zest from a navel orange (see Notes)

8 large pasture-raised egg yolks (150 g)

½ cup (100 g) packed light brown sugar

1 cup (220 ml/225 g) heavy cream

1 tablespoon Pimm's (see Notes)

¼ teaspoon fine sea salt

1. Combine the milk, bananas, and orange zest in a medium, heavy-bottomed lidded pot. Bring to a simmer, uncovered, over medium-high heat, then remove from the heat and place the lid on the pot. Allow the mixture to steep for 20 minutes and then strain.

2. Bring the milk to a scald (just before it boils). Meanwhile, place the egg yolks and sugar in a bowl and whisk until the yolks are pale and the sugar is dissolved.

3. Ladle 1 cup (240 ml) of the hot milk into the egg mixture while whisking. Carefully whisk the tempered egg mixture into the remaining hot milk.

4. Cook the custard over medium heat, stirring constantly with a heatproof spatula, until the mixture reaches 180°F (82°C) and the custard coats the back of a spoon without dripping.

5. Pour the cream into a large bowl. Whisk the mixture into the cream, along with the Pimm's and salt.

6. Chill overnight and then spin according to the manufacturer's directions for your ice cream machine. Store in a container in the freezer to firm further.

NOTES

Use a vegetable peeler to most efficiently remove the zest in strips from a navel orange.

If you do not have Pimm's, any spiced rum works nicely as well.

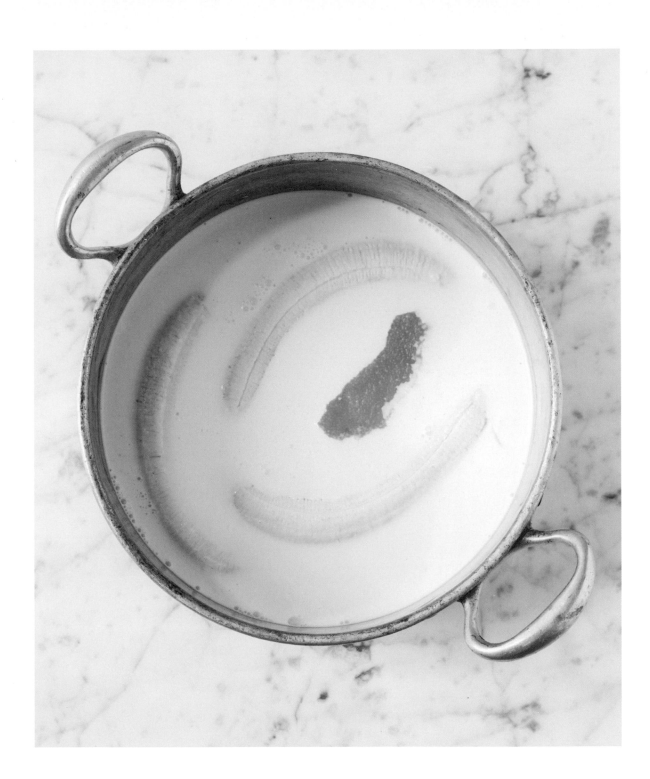

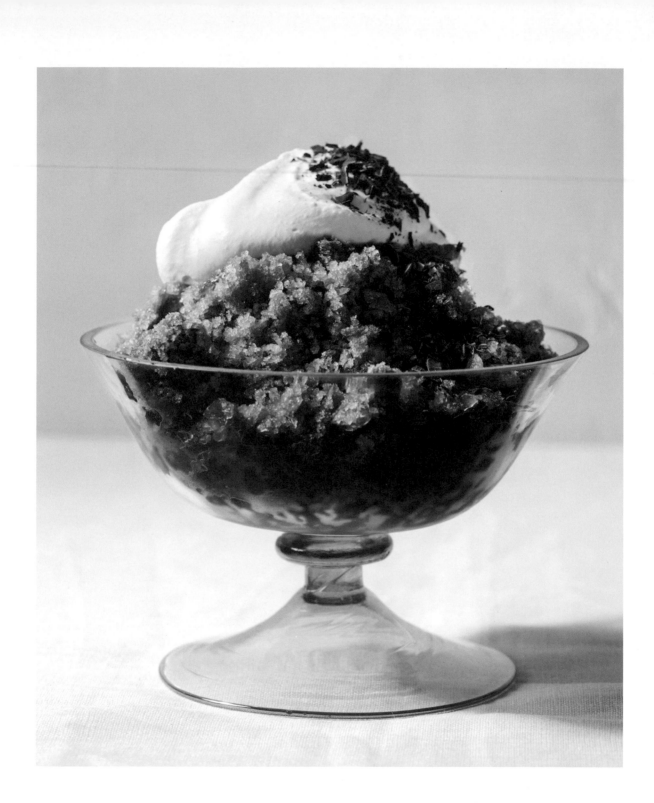

CREAMY CAFÉ GRANITA

Iced coffee with a dollop of fresh cream—that is what this granita evokes. I love espresso granita on its own, for it makes me dream about my wandering through southern Tuscany on a sojourn. A little rocky beach town called Porto Santo Stefano that I stumbled upon had many a gelato and granita stand. My best memory of that trip is after a day at Cala Grande, which required quite a hike to and from the shore, when I sat and watched the sun set while sipping a perfect café granita. A taste of the good life—it's yours to create.

Makes 4 servings

Scant 2 cups (450 ml) brewed strong coffee, warm

½ cup (100 g) organic granulated cane sugar

1 teaspoon fresh lemon juice

Pinch of sea salt

Fresh Whipped Cream (page 245)

Grated chocolate or cocoa powder, optional

1. Combine the coffee, sugar, lemon juice, and salt in a bowl and whisk together until the sugar is dissolved. Alternatively, use a high-powered blender to combine on high speed for 30 seconds.

2. Pour the mixture into a Pyrex casserole dish and place in the freezer and stir every 30 minutes, with a fork or whisk, until frozen. This will take about 2 hours.

3. Using a fork, scrape and further break up the granita.

4. Store the snow in an airtight container in the freezer.

5. When ready to serve, chill small glasses or bowls in the freezer, then place between ½ and 1 cup (75 and 150 g) of the granita in each. Top with a heavy dollop of cream and sprinkle with grated chocolate or cocoa, if desired.

MILKSHAKES

I make a pretty mean milkshake, and I'm not afraid to say it. Years at Max Brenner left me highly skilled in dreaming up concoctions made of chocolate ganache, ice cream, and ice with of course a splash of ice-cold organic whole milk. Since you have some Original Custard on hand (page 217), you have great chocolate always in your pantry, and you know that getting the best milk possible for your every day makes all the difference, I hope you enjoy these shakes as much as I do, and as regularly—even after an elegant soiree.

SCHOOL LUNCH

Makes 1 serving

1 cup (185 g) ice

½ cup (120 g) cold Milk Chocolate Ganache (page 236)

¼ cup (60 g) creamy natural peanut butter

¼ cup (60 ml) ice-cold milk

1½ tablespoons Erma's Strawberry Preserves (page 244)

Blend together all the ingredients in a high-powered blender and serve in a tall glass.

IT'S MY BIRTHDAY

Makes 1 serving

1 cup (185 g) ice

½ cup (120 g) White Chocolate Ganache, cold (page 236)

¼ cup (60 g) Original Custard, frozen (page 217)

¼ cup (60 g) Original Custard, melted (page 217)

1 Classic Shortbread cookie (page 142)

2 tablespoons candied fennel seeds or rainbow sprinkles, plus more to finish

Fresh Whipped Cream (page 245)

1. Blend together all the ingredients, except the whipped cream, in a high-powered blender and serve in a tall glass.

2. Top with the whipped cream and additional candied fennel seeds or sprinkles.

FUDGE BLITZ

Makes 1 serving

1⅓ cups (300 g) Original Custard, frozen (page 217)

½ cup (120 g) Fudge Sauce, cold (page 235), plus more to drizzle

1 ounce (28 g) 75% dark chocolate wafers (Michel Cluizel preferred)

Fresh Whipped Cream (page 245)

1. Blend together the Original Custard, ½ cup (120 g) of the Fudge Sauce, and the chocolate wafers in a high-powered blender and serve in a tall glass.

2. Top with the whipped cream and drizzle with the fudge sauce.

HALVA MILKSHAKE

Makes 1 serving

1⅓ cups (300 g) Original Custard, frozen (page 217)

¼ cup (60 ml) ice-cold whole milk

¼ cup (60 g) Milk Chocolate Ganache, cold (page 236)

¼ cup (60 g) tahini paste

1 tablespoon Original Treacle Sauce (page 234)

Fresh Whipped Cream (page 245)

Halva threads or crushed halva candy

1. Blend together all the ingredients, except the whipped cream and halva, in a high-powered blender and serve in a tall glass.

2. Top with the whipped cream and sprinkle with the halva.

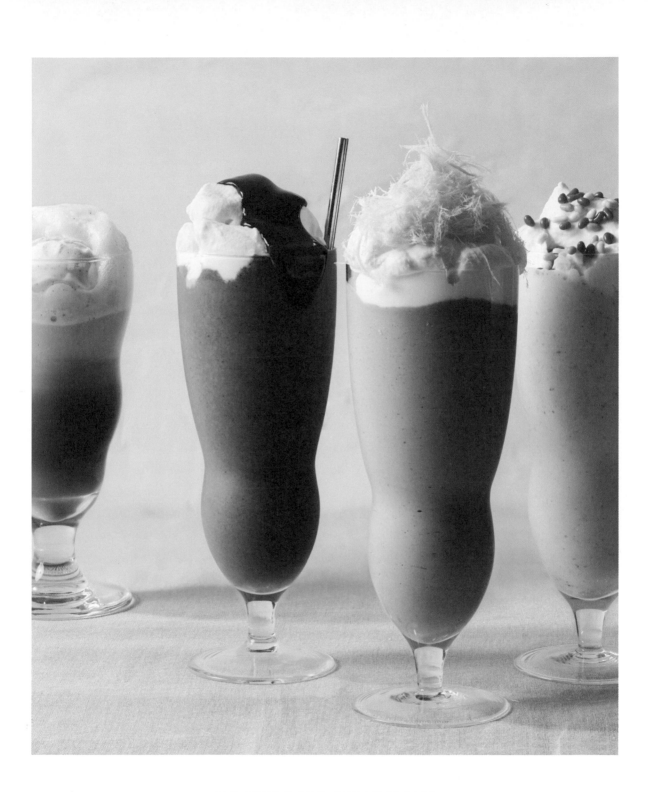

SWEET PANTRY

A lot of baking and making pastry is based on a set of core ingredients, dessert forms (such as cakes, cookies, pies), and "anchor" recipes. *Clean Enough* promotes simplicity in both savory and sweet recipes even when the resulting dish appears more complex. By utilizing anchor recipes for preserves, sauces, curds, and creams across a variety of cookie doughs, blini, cakes, meringues, and ice creams, you are able to leverage these base recipes an endless number of ways. I have a penchant for making such craveable concoctions as my Original Treacle Sauce, Praline Honey, Honey Butter, and the like. These sauces, when sandwiched between cookies, swirled with ice cream, or served simply with a beautiful tray of fruit, have been a part of many memorable dessert moments—and many to come.

Refer to this section as called for throughout the sweet side of the book, or when you want to make a curd or ganache to have on hand so you're prepared when the mood strikes for a Hot Mess or a milkshake. Whip up a batch of truffles that can stand on their own as petite dessert, showcased on your favorite tray, or beautifully packaged as a gift.

The techniques vary throughout this section and many call for emulsification of a substance, which is a simple technique that will serve you well once mastered. Emulsification is an even blend or binding of multiple ingredients and is often best achieved using an immersion stick blender or blender wand. This is explained more in the Tools of the Trade section of the book (page 129).

While you can surely purchase lemon curds, chocolate sauces, and jams at the store, they are almost always exponentially better when you make them by hand. You are able to choose exactly what you put into your next batch of fudge sauce, and in turn get comfortable with how remarkably achievable these recipes are to make.

PRALINE PASTE

I love making my own praline paste. I think that it is one of my favorite condiments of sorts in the sweet world and a minimal labor of love to produce. A good slow roast of hazelnuts ensuring a deep even brown and an eye for a dangerously dark caramel are the secrets to a great praline paste. The flavor is much more pungent than peanut butter, and praline paste is often used as an ingredient rather than on its own.

Makes 2½ cups (600 g)

Olive oil for parchment

2½ cups (340 g) raw hazelnuts, skin on

Scant 1½ cups (280 g) organic granulated cane sugar

1. Preheat the oven to 300°F (150°C) convection. Grease a parchment sheet with the oil and set it aside.

2. Place the hazelnuts in a single layer on a sheet pan and slowly toast in the oven, tossing every 4 to 5 minutes, until golden brown throughout.

3. Remove the hazelnuts from the oven and, wearing rubber gloves, rub the nuts between your hands to remove and discard the skins. Roughly chop the hazelnuts.

4. Place a small, heavy-bottomed saucepan over medium-high heat. Allow the pan to heat and add a tablespoon of the sugar, using a heatproof spatula to swirl and melt.

5. Continue to add the sugar slowly, making sure that each fresh tablespoon melts before adding more. Cook the caramel until it is dark amber, just before it burns. This will happen in under a minute.

6. Immediately add the still-warm chopped hazelnuts to the caramel and scrape out the entire mixture onto the greased parchment sheet, using the spatula.

7. Allow the caramel to cool and harden completely into a brittle.

8. Break up the hazelnut caramel into small pieces and place in a food processor. Grind the brittle, scraping the sides every so often, until it turns into a liquid paste. This will take about 5 minutes.

9. Store in an airtight container at room temperature for up to 2 weeks. You can freeze the praline paste, too, for up to 3 months.

ORIGINAL TREACLE SAUCE

I am fairly certain that this concoction was the result of complete lack of sleep and an odd moment of creativity to feed a fat and sugar craving. It begs to be swirled into Original Custard, tossed with bananas and puddin', or eaten straight from the jar. Flavor abounds.

Makes 3 cups (800 g)

6 or 7 large pasture-raised egg yolks (120 g)

¼ cup (60 ml) + 1 tablespoon organic corn syrup

1 pound (4 sticks/450 g) organic unsalted butter

1 cup + 2 teaspoons (225 g) organic granulated cane sugar

Scant ¾ cup (175 ml/180 g) heavy cream

1 teaspoon fresh lemon juice

1 teaspoon Maldon sea salt flakes

1. Place the egg yolks in a food processor with the ¼ cup (60 ml) corn syrup. Pulse to combine.

2. Place the butter in a medium saucepan over medium-low heat. Once the butter is melted, increase the heat to medium and continue to cook until the milk solids separate and begin to bubble. Cook the butter until the milk solids brown, using a heatproof spatula to scrape the bottom so the butter does not burn.

3. With the food processor running, slowly stream the butter into the yolks. Process to emulsify, then turn the machine off and scrape down the sides.

4. Combine the sugar with the remaining tablespoon of corn syrup in a clean medium saucepan. Add enough water to create a wet sand texture, making sure to keep the sides of the pan wiped clean.

5. Cook the caramel over medium-high heat without stirring, as this will cause the caramel to seize, until it reaches a medium dark amber color.

6. Immediately whisk in the cream and lemon juice.

7. With the food processor running, slowly stream the caramel sauce into the egg mixture. Add the salt last.

8. Store the sauce in an airtight container in the fridge.

9. The sauce can be used warmed, cold, or at room temperature.

FUDGE SAUCE

The difference between fudge and ganache lies in cocoa powder and any additional sugar beyond what is already in your chocolate. When I say *cocoa*, I am referring to deliciously dark cocoa brut powder that in its "uncooked" form could potentially taste chalky. When you cook cocoa in a milk mixture, the texture and flavor smooths out. With the addition of tangy brown sugar and glossy corn syrup as well as a combination of milk and dark chocolate, you end up with an ultraglossy rich fudge sauce that is the secret to the Fudge Blitz milkshake (page 230) and will be a staple on your ice cream sundae bar. Serve this sauce warm or hot when used as a sauce, or cold for milkshakes and truffles.

Makes 5 cups (1.3 kg)

2¼ cups + 1 tablespoon (580 ml/600 g) heavy cream

¾ cup + 1 tablespoon (195 ml/200 g) whole milk

¾ cup (160 g) packed light brown sugar

½ cup (60 g) extra brut cocoa powder

2 tablespoons + 2 teaspoons organic corn syrup

8½ ounces (240 g) 70% dark chocolate wafers (Michel Cluizel preferred)

5½ ounces (160 g) milk chocolate wafers (Michel Cluizel preferred)

3 tablespoons (40 g) organic unsalted butter

1. Combine the cream, milk, sugar, cocoa powder, and corn syrup in a medium saucepan. Whisk well to combine.

2. Bring the mixture to a boil over medium heat and cook, whisking, for 10 minutes. This mixture is viscous and can easily burn on the bottom, so watch it carefully.

3. After 10 minutes, remove the sauce from the heat and whisk in the chocolate wafers and butter.

4. Transfer the sauce to a tall, narrow container and emulsify, using an immersion stick blender fully submerged so as to not allow in air bubbles.

5. Allow the sauce to cool and then store in the fridge until ready to use.

VARIATIONS

Add spices to this sauce to change up the flavor. Licorice powder, cinnamon, and cardamom work well.

M/D/W GANACHE

Basic ganache generally requires equal parts chocolate to heavy cream, emulsified until glossy and smooth. In this case, the liquid has been altered, as dark chocolate contains more cocoa solids, milk chocolate less, and white chocolate no cocoa solids at all! By varying the amount of liquid, you end up with a consistent end product of smooth and creamy Ganache. Use this Ganache for all of your milkshake desires, as an easy glaze on a cake, or to coat or fill cookie sandwiches.

Makes 15 servings (approximately 2¼ pounds/1 kg)

MILK CHOCOLATE

1½ cups (360 ml/375 g) heavy cream

¼ cup + 2 tablespoons (90 ml) whole milk

23 ounces (670 g) milk chocolate wafers (Michel Cluizel preferred)

DARK CHOCOLATE

Scant 1½ cups (350 ml/360 g) heavy cream

½ cup (120 ml) whole milk

17 ounces (500 g) 70% dark chocolate wafers (Michel Cluizel preferred)

WHITE CHOCOLATE

1 cup (240 ml/250 g) heavy cream

¼ cup + 1 tablespoon (75 g) whole milk

23 ounces (670 g) white chocolate wafers (Michel Cluizel preferred)

1. Place the cream and milk in a medium saucepan over medium heat until it comes to a simmer. Meanwhile, place the chocolate wafers in a medium heatproof bowl.

2. Pour the hot cream over the chocolate wafers and allow to sit for 2 minutes to melt the chocolate. Then stir together from the center, using a heatproof spatula.

3. Transfer the mixture to a tall, narrow container and, using an immersion stick blender, emulsify, keeping the wand completely submerged so as to avoid air bubbles.

4. Pour the Ganache into shallow storage containers and place at room temperature to set for 8 hours.

5. Store in an airtight container in the fridge for up to 2 weeks.

———

NOTE

I chill this Ganache in the fridge as I primarily use it for fillings and milkshakes!

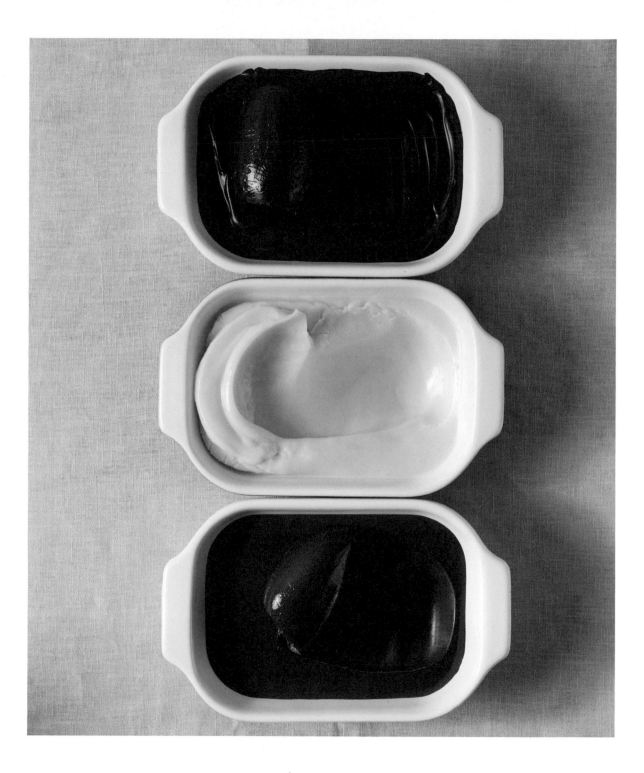

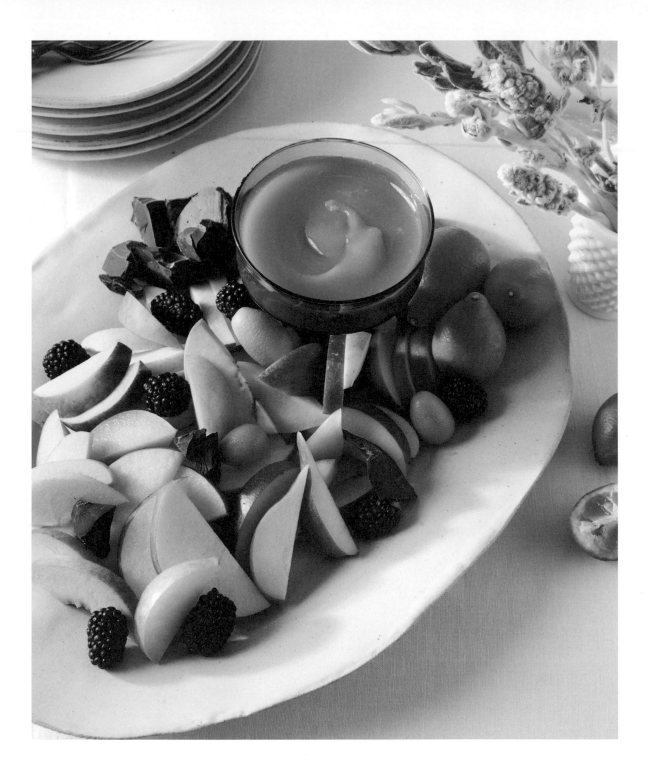

HONEY BUTTER

The simple act of browning high-quality butter to a deep nuttiness and then emulsifying in honey nuanced with your favorite flavor—be it lavender, clover, or orange blossom—results in a taffy-like spread that will become a pantry staple. Warm honey butter to drizzle on a cake or ice cream. Spread honey butter in between shortbreads to create Biancas (page 145). Dip fresh fruit in room-temperature honey butter for a perfect conversational dessert. Roll cold honey butter into mini truffles and coat with dark chocolate for last-minute truffle treats.

Makes 2 cups (675 g)

½ pound (2 sticks/225 g) organic
  unsalted butter

1 pound (450 g) local honey

½ teaspoon Maldon sea salt flakes

1. Place the butter in a medium saucepan and melt over medium-low heat. Once the butter is melted, increase the heat to medium and carefully brown the milk solids. The butter will foam and brown flecks will appear. Stir, using a nonstick spatula, being sure to scrape the bottom of the pan.

2. As soon as the butter browns, whisk in the honey. Bring the mixture to a simmer and immediately turn off the heat.

3. Transfer the mixture to a tall container, add the salt, and, using a stick immersion blender, blend until opaque, taffy-like, and emulsified.

4. Store the honey butter in an airtight container in the fridge for up to 2 weeks.

CREAM CHEESE FROSTING

Υou could eat this off a shoe, without judgment.

Makes 4 cups (900 g)

22 ounces (675 g) cream cheese, at
room temperature

1½ cups (3 sticks/340 g) organic
unsalted butter, room temperature

2¾ cups + 1 tablespoon (340 g)
confectioners' sugar, sifted

1 teaspoon pure vanilla extract

1 teaspoon fine sea salt

1. Place the cream cheese in a stand mixer fitted with the whisk attachment. Paddle on low speed. Add the butter and continue to paddle on low speed.

2. Add the confectioners' sugar gradually while the mixer is running on low speed.

3. Add the vanilla and sea salt.

4. Increase the speed to high and mix for 30 seconds to incorporate all ingredients well, until the frosting is light and just whipped. Whip too far and you will get hard, lumpy frosting, which you cannot eat on a shoe.

5. Store the frosting at room temperature if using that day. Store in the fridge in an airtight container for later use, up to 1 week.

***

NOTES

Cream cheese frosting should be made on low speed; this is how you avoid lumps!

Room-temperature products will also help you avoid butter or cream cheese lumps.

Paddle the cold frosting on low speed to reconstitute prior to use.

CHOCOLATE BAR FROSTING

There are cake-first people and frosting-first people. No matter who you are, I dare you to avoid eating it all before you frost your cake, let alone eat it.

Makes 3 cups (600 g) whipped

8 ounces (225 g) 64% semisweet chocolate wafers (Michel Cluizel preferred)

3½ ounces (75 g) milk chocolate wafers (Michel Cluizel preferred)

1¼ cups (1 stick + 4 tablespoons/ 300 g) organic unsalted butter, softened

½ teaspoon Maldon sea salt flakes

1. Melt the dark and milk chocolate in a glass bowl in the microwave until liquid is warm but not too hot. Stir together well to combine.

2. Place the butter in a stand mixer fitted with the paddle attachment. Paddle on high speed for 4 minutes.

3. Stream the melted chocolate into the whipping butter, scraping down, then paddle in the salt.

4. Store in an airtight container at room temperature for up to 2 weeks.

NOTE

If the frosting is too liquid, let it cool on the counter slightly and whip to add air before frosting your cake. Alternatively, you can place the frosting in the fridge, and it will start to solidify around the edges. Scrape the solidified chocolate into the center of the bowl and paddle to aerate and combine.

CREAMY LEMON CURD

Tangy and ready for a slathering on a scone, folding into whipped cream, or layering between some of my favorite cakes. The portion of orange juice brightens the curd and acts as a faux Meyer lemon flavor. Make sure to strain this using a fine-mesh strainer.

Makes 4 cups (1 kg)

6 large pasture-raised eggs (300 g)

5 large pasture-raised egg yolks (100 g)

1 cup + 2 teaspoons (225 g) organic granulated cane sugar

2 teaspoons grated lemon zest

Pinch of grated orange zest

¾ cup + 1 tablespoon (195 ml) fresh lemon juice

¼ cup + 1 tablespoon (75 ml) fresh orange juice

6 tablespoons (90 g) organic unsalted butter, softened

Pinch of fine sea salt

1. Fill a saucepan with 2 inches (5 cm) of water and heat to a simmer. Have ready a metal or glass bowl that can fit on top without touching the water. (This will create a double boiler that produces indirect heat, to slowly cook the curd.)

2. Place the eggs, yolks, sugar, and lemon and orange zest in the bowl and whisk until dissolved.

3. Place the bowl atop the saucepan of simmering water and stream in the lemon and orange juice, whisking until the mixture reaches 180°F (82°C).

4. Using an immersion blender or a high-powered blender, blend the curd with the butter and salt until glossy and emulsified.

5. Strain the mixture, using a fine-mesh strainer, into a shallow pan or glass dish.

6. Cover with plastic wrap and place in the fridge to chill for 4 hours or overnight. This curd can be frozen or stored in the fridge for 1 week prior to use.

CANDIED ORANGE PEEL

Simpler than you may have realized, orange peel adds flavor—sweet, aromatic, and slightly bitter—to recipes.

Makes 1 cup (150 g)

3 oranges

1 cup (215 g) organic granulated cane sugar

1. Using a vegetable peeler, remove the orange peel from the oranges, leaving any white pith on the fruit. Place the peel in cold water and let sit for 10 minutes to remove any bitter flavor.

2. Combine the sugar and a ½ cup (120 ml) water in a small saucepan and heat over medium heat to dissolve the sugar fully.

3. Drain the orange peel and place in a small container. Pour the sugar syrup over the peel and place in the fridge to cool overnight.

4. Store in the fridge for up to 1 month. To use the peel, drain from the syrup and dice into a few small pieces.

EARL GREY RAISINS

Why would you plump raisins in plain water when you can add the flavor and aroma of tea? A new ritual is born.

Makes 1½ cups (200 g)

2 Earl Grey tea bags

2 tablespoons honey or regular molasses

1 teaspoon fresh lemon juice

1 cup (150 g) dark raisins

1. Boil 1 cup (240 ml) water and combine with tea bags, honey, and lemon juice in a heatproof bowl. Allow to steep for 5 minutes.

2. Place the raisins in another heatproof bowl and strain the liquid over the raisins. Allow to soak for 1 hour.

3. Store in the refrigerator in the soaking liquid for up to 2 weeks.

___

VARIATION

Chamomile Raisins: Replace the tea bags with 2 tablespoons dried chamomile flowers and the dark raisins with golden, and use 2 tablespoons honey instead of molasses.

ERMA'S STRAWBERRY PRESERVES

Erma was my mother's beloved aunt. They were kindred spirits and Mom cherished her relationship with Erma as they were both independent with a steady hand for crafts and the homemade. The filing cabinet in my basement was always stocked with tall Ball jars of Erma's Strawberry Preserves. I am not talking pulverized jam here. I am talking syrupy whole strawberries that you could smash on top of a great piece of toast (or cheesecake, for that matter). A glossy, vibrant, and juicy nod to early summer all year round.

Makes 3 cups (700 g)

4 cups (550 g) fresh strawberries, hulled

1 cup (215 g) + 2 teaspoons organic granulated cane sugar

2 teaspoons pectin

1 tablespoon fresh lemon juice

Pinch of fine sea salt

1. Combine the strawberries and 1 cup (215 g) of the sugar in a large bowl. Stir to coat and allow to macerate for 4 hours at room temperature.

2. Place the strawberries and their liquid in a medium, heavy-bottomed saucepan over medium heat and cook, stirring with a whisk, for 4 minutes.

3. Combine the pectin with the remaining 2 teaspoons sugar in a small bowl, then, whisking constantly, shake the pectin mixture into the strawberries. Continue to whisk for 5 minutes to gel the preserves, whisking in the lemon juice and salt in the last minute of cooking. The goal is to cook the strawberries quickly, preserving their bright red juicy color and flavor.

4. Pour the preserves into sterilized jars or storage containers (see Notes) and allow the jars to cool.

___

NOTES

To can the preserves, sterilize a screw-top or flip-top canning jar in the dishwasher or a pot of boiling water. Fill the jar with the hot preserves and secure with a sterilized lid while hot. Bring a large pot of water to a boil. Insert the sealed jar and boil for 5 minutes. Remove the jar with tongs and allow to cool. These preserves will keep for over 3 months, if they last that long.

If you don't want to can the preserves, simply store the jam in an airtight container in the fridge for a few weeks, or the freezer for a year.

There will be whole strawberry pieces in your preserves. You can easily blend chilled preserves to make a smoother jam.

MASCARPONE CREAM

Don't eat all of this before you serve it! Perfect for Pan di Spagna (page 156), in dirt cake (see page 214), and simply as a dip for a bowl of fresh fruit.

Makes 4 cups (750 g) whipped

13 ounces (375 g) mascarpone cheese

1½ cups (360ml/375 g) heavy cream

⅓ cup (45 g) confectioners' sugar

½ teaspoon orange zest

½ teaspoon vanilla bean seeds

1. Place the mascarpone in the bowl of a mixer fitted with the whisk attachment.

2. Whip on low, streaming in the cream slowly to prevent clumping.

3. Add the confectioners' sugar, orange zest, and vanilla and continue to whip until stiff peaks form.

4. Store in the fridge until ready to use, for up to 6 hours.

FRESH WHIPPED CREAM

An Enough staple.

Makes 1½ cups (225 g)

Scant 1 cup (220 ml/225 g) organic full-fat heavy cream

1 tablespoon granulated cane sugar

½ teaspoon pure vanilla extract

1. Combine all the ingredients in a cold, stainless-steel bowl and whisk by hand until soft peaks form.

2. Store the soft cream in the fridge until ready to serve.

VARIATION

Elderflower Cream: Add ½ cup (115 g) crème fraîche to the heavy cream before whipping. Whip to soft peaks and fold in 1½ tablespoons St-Germain elderflower liqueur.

ACKNOWLEDGMENTS

WHERE WOULD I BE WITHOUT YOU?

Tied to many of my stories and this book is my remarkable mother, Janet. She was the first person to tell me that if I wanted to leave college and become a pastry chef, that I wasn't crazy, but that I'd better be successful. I listened. When I wanted to move to California, on a whim, she was there. Through the happy highs and tearful lows, my mom has been on speed dial. She is wise and kind with a directness that I gratefully possess. One of the most naturally glamorous women I know, who is never without her lipstick, she shines bright. I owe her everything (including a villa in Italy).

Sherry Yard, at first a maternal figure, then a mentor, and now someone I would call a true and dear friend. I adore this woman. I am grateful for the trail that she has blazed for women. Chefs, pastry chefs, and business leaders alike. As a woman working and owning her creativity and style, Sherry was one of the firsts. Never have I seen this woman deterred. We have an understanding, or a knowing that is very much mutual, something I have always recognized and undoubtedly cherish. Monkey Girl.

Katherine Sacks, one of the first people to intercept me as a young pastry cook arriving for my first day of work at Spago, all the way through life, straight to this book. I apparently tried to steal her name when we first began working together, hence

the solidification from Kat (old me) to Katzie. Kat is a talent beyond even her own realization. Creative, intelligent, hardworking, and passionate about all aspects of food culture. Her deep dive into and respect for Japanese culture and cuisine has been fascinating to witness, and I cannot wait to see how it will continue to bear fruit. This book would not have been possible without her. Her dedication to preparing, styling, scaling, and being a figure of strength for the creation of these photos moved me. I look forward to returning the favor.

I have no direct place to begin with Amy Harsch. Supportive in every moment from a young girl to now. Amy knows how to do it all well, with a specific grace and integrity. The sweet portion of this book would not have existed without her generosity and taste for a well-designed functional kitchen and selfless act of love.

Keren's eye, nobody has it. My favorite curly-haired, chocolate-loving woman, who brought so much kindness and discernment to these images. She is honest and encouraging, with a talent for look, feel, and texture that you cannot learn.

My family. My sister, Rebecca; brother, Matthew; and honorary brother, Peter. To be so lucky to have a team of people who believe in you, and who you believe in as well. Thank you for your patience and support during this endeavor. Emma, Sean, and Margie, I hope I have made Robbie proud. To the entirety of the Guys, Hamiltons, McKelvies, Clearys, and beyond. The encouragement, love, and support throughout this process produced a dynamic force. Each and every one of you mean the world.

The dynamic duo of Jennifer Kurdyla and Sarah Smith. To have an editor and an agent who understand your point of view, internalize it, and express it in their own way is Clean Enough. Sarah's commitment to not making this a book about clean food, a dessert bible, or a collection of thoughts about mindfulness and self-care, but rather a collective approach to a life well lived is why we can all be Clean Enough. Jennifer's remarkable patience and ability to synthesize run-on thoughts, actions, and sentences have no match; my gratitude for her continues to grow by the day. Sarah Smith, the other Sarah, for designing an incredibly beautiful book and putting up with trying to understand the inner workings of my creative brain.

To the women in my life: Sarah, Samantha, Anna, Puja, Rebecca, Andrea, Rachel, Tarin, Jacquie, Callie, Amanda, Berkley, Michelle, Brianna, Mary-Kate, Alicia, Ali, Megan, Leigh . . . Every. Single. One. Of. You. You are enough, you are brilliant, and your unique gifts and friendship have both inspired and challenged this work, an extension of myself. I am both embraced and better because of *all* of you.

To Equinox and Furthermore, and everyone who makes up this engine of thinkers and doers. These high-performance individuals continue to keep me motivated to execute and follow through with all of life's projects. A powerful group embodying movement, nutrition, and regeneration both personally and professionally. Collectively the people I am grateful to be surrounded by take a stand that to live and perform better you must individually be better. To the partnerships cultivated through the Equinox halo, every smoothie, tea, product, and perspective is what keeps me committed.

To my culinary school, which will forever be the French Culinary Institute, now the International Culinary Center. The education, community, and ongoing support that I am able to contribute to, enjoy, and be a part of is unique. Chef Jurgen, Jansen Chan, Ron-Ben Israel, and the rest of the community carrying the torch of Dorothy Cann-Hamilton keep my sweet spirit alive and bright.

To my universe, all of equal importance. My family of friends held together by the Clarkes and one Christopher Lee, the most brilliant group of misfits to call your own, and the new generation led by Remy, Ali, and Charlotte. Michael and Erin and the RYE family, there would be no Banana Luscious without all of you. My Max Brenner posse, forever tied together by incredibly chocolate-covered experiences. Michel Cluizel and Jacques Dahan, your generosity has coated this book in milk, dark, and white. To everyone tied to this work in the present, past, and into the future: Thank you.

And finally to all of my healers, followers of the moon, and those with one constant: love.

INDEX

INDEX

ABOUT THE AUTHOR

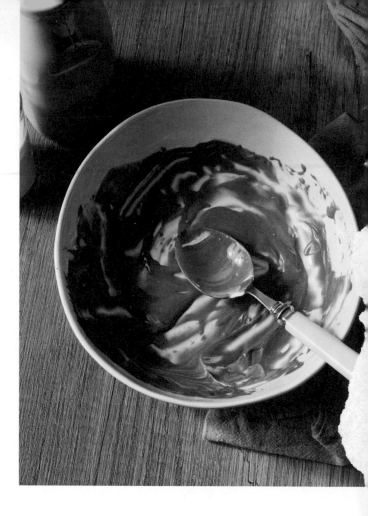

Katzie Guy-Hamilton is a nationally recognized pastry chef and creative, now the food and beverage director at the luxury fitness brand Equinox. Prior to entering the high-performance world of wellness, Katzie ran all Global Food and Beverage and Innovation for the indulgent chocolate brand Max Brenner International. She ran the pastry departments at Grand Hyatt's New York flagship in Grand Central and the celebrated pastry program at New York's trendsetting Ace Hotel. She trained in California under pastry maven Sherry Yard at Wolfgang Puck's Spago Beverly Hills. She is a graduate of the French Culinary Institute and recipient of its Outstanding Alumni of the Year for 2011. Katzie's talents earned her a spot on Season Two of the television cooking competition *Top Chef: Just Desserts*. She was named one of the Top Ten Pastry Chefs in America by *Dessert Professional Magazine* in 2014.

Katzie teaches healthy cooking at Goal4Kids in Harlem and cochairs October Ball, benefitting the Catholic Big Sisters and Big Brothers Organization. She embodies the concept of living mindfully in the middle and is a certified health coach by the Institute for Integrative Nutrition. Katzie's mission is to inspire others to learn their happiest selves through clean eating, delicious indulgences, and a collective approach to integrative health. Katzie has appeared on Fox Network, Martha Stewart Radio, CBS, Food Network, Bravo TV, and internationally, in Japanese, Australian, and Korean media, as well as in various print and digital publications.